BALANCING
YOUR
BODY

BALANCING
YOUR
BODY

A Self-help Approach to
Rolfing Movement

MARY BOND

Healing Arts Press
Rochester, Vermont

Healing Arts Press
One Park Street
Rochester, Vermont 05767
www.InnerTraditions.com

Note to the reader: This book is intended as an informational guide. The remedies, approaches, and techniques described herein are meant to supplement, and not to be a substitute for, professional medical care or treatment. They should not be used to treat a serious ailment without prior consultation with a qualified healthcare professional.

The word Rolfing is a service mark of The ROLF INSTITUTE of Structural Integration.

LIBRARY OF CONGRESS CATALOGING-IN-PUBLICATION DATA
Bond, Mary, 1942–
    Balancing your body : a self-help approach to Rolfing Movement / Mary Bond.
        p.   cm.
    Includes index.
    ISBN 978-0-89281-642-2
    1. Rolfing.   I. Title.
RC489.R64B66   1996
615.8'22—dc20   96-24187
                                                                                CIP

Printed and bound in the United States.

10 9 8 7

Text design by Virginia L. Scott

Illustrations by Barbara Mindell
This book was typeset in Berkeley Oldstyle with Carolus as the display typeface.

Healing Arts Press is a division of Inner Traditions International.

CONTENTS

RULES OF THE GRAVITY GAME

It's seventh grade and the day for posture evaluations. You line up outside the nurse's office, grateful for your reprieve from that history quiz. Inside, the nurse draws dots down your back with a marker, and pointing to a chart of spinal curvatures, explains the dire consequences of scoliosis (lateral curvature of the spine). The scoliosis threat is exciting for a day or two—there's talk that Terri Dawson has it and might have to wear a brace. For the most part, though, posture is a boring topic that is soon blithely forgotten. Your sophistication mimics the images you see in magazines, and "standing up straight" doesn't look cool.

Traveling forward in time now, let's visit your fiftieth high school reunion. Do you look and feel as vital, supple, and dignified as you'd like to? If not, why not? Many things affect your body in between seventh grade and your seventieth birthday—diet, exercise, work, play, love, and luck, to name a few. Another important factor is your attitude toward your body. Is it just something to be decorated or camouflaged, a mere vehicle to transport you from one experience to the next?

Most of us take our bodies for granted. At the beginning of our game of life we're dealt a number of "selves," like cards or Monopoly properties. There's the mental/intellectual self—the one who goes to college and becomes a CEO; there's the emotional self who falls in and out of love and cries at movies; and there's the spiritual self who seeks meaning in religion or peace in meditation. The physical self, the body, is relegated to carrying the other selves to job and church and dance floor. It's taken for granted until one day, in the middle of the game, the body self prevents one of the other selves from making a move.

Your body's "shape" is not just its appearance but its ability to move you energetically and gracefully through your days. And your shape begins to be determined long before that nurse's hasty appraisal of your posture. Very early we begin to shape ourselves by modeling the people around us, usually our parents and siblings. We unconsciously imitate their rhythms, postures, gestures, and tensions. These people comprise our known world—we need to feel close to them, so we do as they do.

Come adolescence, we generally overlay our familial, acquired, movement patterns with the gestures of our friends, with the postures of our heroes, with the stance of our rebellion. Later, as we enter adulthood, we model images of accomplishment and success. In today's media-rich world, we're increasingly tempted to assume shapes we see outside ourselves.

Though women's roles in our society have begun to change in recent decades, the media continue to portray women's bodies according to outmoded physical ideals. Fashion offers women two alternatives. One is the low-slung model's stance—pelvis under, chest withdrawn, and head forward—a combination of passiveness and seduction. The other more assertive and extroverted stance has breasts and head high, back arched and "buns" up. Both stances suggest woman is man's sexual adjunct. A woman is rarely portrayed standing on her own two feet, except in a kind of mannish defiance. As women's changing roles and collective self-concept become more defined and secure, the media's portrayal of women's bodies will change.

As for men: you poor fellows are trained from infancy to "keep it all together," to project an image of rock-hard stability and stoicism. For men to be expressive with their bodies has been a sign of weakness in our culture, mobility of spine or pelvis a signal of effeminacy. Elvis Presley introduced a measure of freedom within the confines of the entertainment industry—so as long as you're making music, guys, it's okay to move your hips. As men's roles change, the media begin to portray men in more relaxed postures.

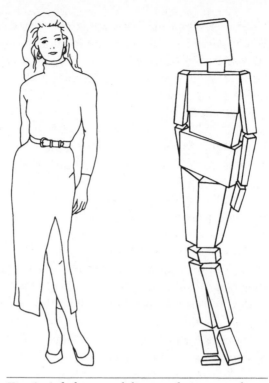

Fig. 1: A fashion model's casual grace masks an imbalanced structure and unstable stance.

But for every man who looks at home in his body, there remains an army of stiff upper lips and girded loins.

Besides these familial and cultural models, what else determines your shape? Accidents, trauma, illness—all those life stresses leave you depleted, less whole than you were before. Remember that skiing accident? the whiplash? the time you caught your heel and slipped on the stairs? Ever since, you have felt just slightly off-kilter, not so agile or free in your body as before. And what about all that weight you gained after your lover walked out, the long months of depression and therapy before you regained your self-esteem? You lost the weight eventually, but you never quite recovered your old sense of lightness and ease.

And then, of course, there's your job. Maybe you spend long hours in front of a computer terminal. Or you're a dental hygienist, bending over and twisting to peer into patients' mouths. Or you brace a telephone against your shoulder as you take down messages. Or you carry heavy equipment to and from a construction site. We use our bodies in an endless variety of ways, and few of us come home at night without some complaint about the physical effects of the day's activities.

Our bodies must be made of soft plastic to be so easily molded by role models, fashion, trauma, and occupational hazards—by life in general. As we approach middle age, when the plastic has become less pliable, our bodies start attracting our attention in a new way. We stop bouncing back. We call it "getting old," and for its early appearance, we blame the luck of the draw. We'd give anything for our bodies to feel good again, to regain the freedom and ease we once had.

Believe it or not, this can be done. The first step in this direction is to revamp our attitudes about what the body is. Instead of regarding it as a handicap, we need to consider that the body is shaped by the manner in which we live in it. Since our bodies are so responsive, perhaps *we* bear *them* some responsibility.

Suppose that instead of being a card you're dealt at the beginning of your lifegame, your body is actually the field where the game is played. Maybe the Good Book had the right idea—your body is a temple, the moving architecture in which you dwell.* Thinking of it that way, your body does a lot more than just disguise you, contain you, and carry you around. Every aspect of it expresses you. And whatever happens to it is integral to you.

All Fall Down

Every object in the universe is motivated by gravity. Newton's universal law of gravity—a main tenet in the field of physics—states that all objects in the universe attract all other objects in the universe. The force of attraction is greater or smaller depending on size and distance, but the attraction is nonetheless present everywhere.

This force that binds us to the earth and binds the stars and planets together is generally unrecognized as a factor in our physical

---

*I Corinthians 6:19–20.

well-being. Yet, since our bodies are physical structures, they're subject to the same physical laws as any other structure on the planet. A structure that is not in a balanced relationship to the pull of gravity will topple over due to the immensely greater magnitude of the earth than of any object upon it. Gravity may be temporarily defied by other factors—by mechanical energy, by speed, by balance— but when push comes to shove, down you go.

How we move, with or against gravity's influence, amounts to a game with gravity. Or perhaps it is rather a game that gravity plays with us. How graciously we let gravity play on and through the body's field largely determines our shape as septuagenarians.

Think about the last time you tripped over something. At the moment you were about to fall, you had several choices—to brace yourself with tension, to relax totally and surrender to whatever experience gravity had in store for you, or any variation of response that lay in between these two extremes.

Our instinct is usually the first choice—to brace with tension against the fall. We try to keep the temple at status quo. When the earth moves, literally or figuratively, we temporarily defy gravity by buttressing the body with tension. If this temporary bracing holds long after the fall, the body accepts it as permanent support, and the pattern of compensation is rigidified. Since this tension is not integral to the structure, it leaves the body unbalanced and vulnerable.

A second jolt can cause worse damage and often seems uncannily aimed right at the site of repair. About the time you stop favoring the foot with the broken toe, you sprain your ankle.

Seismological engineers know that structural soundness in a building requires a mobile foundation and flexible supports. Rigidity spells disaster in an earthquake. This is no less true for the human body. The more flexible and resilient is your body, the more secure is its relation to gravity and the more enduring its vitality.

A Metaphor for Love

We fight gravity for emotional reasons as well as for purely physical ones. Emotional or physical abuse, loss, abandonment, rejection—all of these correspond to an emotional "fall," and our response to them is to protect our feelings by tightening our bodies. Curiously, when the emotional rug is pulled out from under us, our

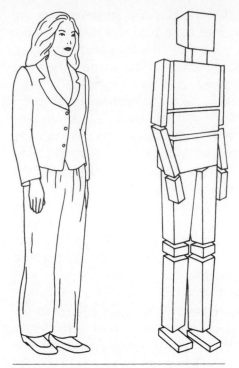

Figure 2: Balance in gravity looks and feels peaceful.

response is just as physical as if the rug were real. Could it be that our physical experience of gravity is in some way a template for our emotional experience of security?

Suppose, instead of fighting gravity, we let it support us. Imagine how it might feel to have gravity as your partner rather than your adversary. Your first experience of support was in infancy, when your parents' love embraced you both physically and emotionally. Throughout your life you've had other experiences of support—from friends, a respected teacher, a lucky gamble in the stock market. Remember how your body felt at those times: balanced, grounded, secure, buoyant, flexible, expansive, graceful, easy, free. When your body is balanced in relation to gravity, these same physical sensations are present. Gravity is nurturing you, and it feels very much like being loved.

Christian symbolism reflects the law of gravitation with the Star of Bethlehem—gravity heralds the birth of love. The star's attraction for the earth symbolizes the love that binds us to one another as human beings and gives us our first feeling of being supported in the physical universe.

When we lose the assurance of support and begin bracing ourselves against life's buffeting, we lose our original relationship with gravity. We stop feeling supported physically, and we stop feeling loved. When we vie with gravity, for whatever reason, we restrict our capacity to fully embody and freely express love.

Emotionally based defiance of gravity leaves tracks of tension in the body, embedded gestures of rage, grief, fear, and pain. We may not be conscious of these tracks in our flesh, and they may not be visible to the untrained eye. But they underlie our communication with one another and influence our handling of the world. They change the blueprint for the temple. For example, you pick up a cup of tea in a way that seems utterly ordinary. But the way you use your arm and shoulder is patterned by a moment of impatience your mother had when you were three. As she yanked you away from the playground, there was a moment of searing pain, confusion, and loss of trust. Ever afterward, free use of your arm is hampered by a protective cringing gesture that you're not even aware of. It is automatic, even when you reach out to embrace another.

Restoring Your Relationship with Gravity

So what's to be done? Do we have to be prisoners of the flesh? Or are there ways to restore the flesh to its original vitality and erase its imprint of pain?

This book suggests that one way is to restore the sensation of support through awareness of gravitational imbalances in the body and release of the tensions that preserve them. When the physical tensions release, emotional components also let go, clearing a path through the body where both gravity and love can travel unimpeded.

Rolfing* and Rolfing Movement

Ida P. Rolf, Ph.D., was the first person to articulate the idea that gravity could support human structures. She called it a "more human use of human beings." Starting in the 1930s, Dr. Rolf developed a ten-step series of physical manipulations that she called Structural Integration. She worked from the premise that bodies were plastic—if they could be molded into imbalanced shapes by gravity, then they could be restored to balance through human touch. By the 1960s, her method had acquired notoriety and its popular name, Rolfing.[†]

Dr. Rolf recognized that if people who had been Rolfed didn't learn to use their bodies differently, they often reverted to their original imbalances and lost the benefits of the treatment. In the sixties and seventies, Rolfer Dorothy Nolte and dancer Judith Aston developed a series of self-help exercises for structural transformation that was effective independent of the Rolfing program.[‡] Numerous other Rolfers and movement specialists have since contributed to the evolution of what we now call Rolfing Movement.[§]

Rolfing Movement combines touch and verbal communication to direct the student's awareness to internal sensations of tension. Using hands and words, the Rolfing Movement teacher assists the student to release the tensions and guides her to discover sensations of being and moving in harmony with gravity. Once a student has learned new patterns in basic activities such as breathing and simple joint movement, she applies the same principles to the activities of daily living—sitting and standing, walking and running, reaching and pushing, working and playing.

Rolfing Movement is much more than lessons in good posture or movement efficiency. If you change your posture superficially, it doesn't feel authentic. Try it right now. Obey that old admonition to hold your shoulders back. It is an effort to do that, isn't it?

---

* The word *Rolfing* is a service mark of The ROLF INSTITUTE of Structural Integration.
† See the bibliography for titles relating to Rolfing.
‡ See the appendix for information regarding Dorothy Nolte's "Structural Awareness" and Judith Aston's "Aston Patterning" programs.
§ Gael Ohlgren, Heather Wing, Vivian Jaye, Jane Harrington, and Megan James have all made major contributions to the development of Rolfing Movement.

And it doesn't feel like the "real you." When you arbitrarily change a body shape or gesture at the surface of the skin, it's like putting on a costume. Or to use the "temple" analogy, it's like restoring the outside of a building without renovating the framing, plumbing, and wiring.

Rolfing Movement takes you on a journey into the blueprint of your structure. Memories of forgotten accidents or emotional stress often surface and resolve as a result of the deep physical awareness. With physical ease and balance come feelings of centeredness, authenticity, and freedom of expression. When structure is changed by these methods, the result feels like a new body, with the real you freed at last from the inside out.

Winning the Gravity Game

This book is an introduction to the basic concepts and teaching methods of Rolfing Movement. Two of the basic concepts we'll be exploring are *stationary* and *moving balance*. Integral to both is the sensation of *gravitational support*.

Rolfers and Rolfing Movement teachers evoke support in three arenas. The first is the *base of support*. This involves the body's foundation—feet, ankles, knees, hips, and pelvis. The second type of support is the body's *dimensionality*—the relationships of width, depth, and length that promote or diminish balanced form. Structural support requires the dimensional balance of front and back, right and left, top and bottom.

The last aspect of support is what we call the *core* of the structure. Anatomically, the core involves the musculature closest to the center of the body. This is where the memory of past traumatic experiences seems to be held and where bracing against pain and anxiety takes place.* Tension in the core places stress on the periphery of the structure, undermining both dimension and foundation. For moment-to-moment centering, the core needs to be flexible and resilient.

In addition to constant support, moving balance requires *fluidity* and *congruency*. Fluidity is the flowing, graceful movement

---

*Hunt, Valerie V., et al. *A Study of Structural Integration from Neuromuscular, Energy Field, and Emotional Approaches* (Unpublished Report), 6.

quality of world-class athletes and dancers. Flexibility is part of it, as is coordination. Fluidity is present when a movement in any part of the body creates an integrated ripple of response throughout the whole.

Congruency indicates integration of movement. The whole body acts in concert—no part hangs back or moves at odds with the rest. You'll observe this trait in the most charismatic leaders and entertainers.

These concepts appear throughout the book as ongoing themes, explored in the contexts of various regions of the body. Dimension, for example, is a theme of the chapter on breathing (chapter 2) and is explored again in the chapter on balancing the two sides of the body (chapter 8).

You may be interested in Rolfing Movement for any number of reasons. Perhaps you've recently had some structural bodywork and are looking for ways to enhance your experience. Or maybe you picked up this book simply for cosmetic reasons. If that's the case, you may get more than you bargained for. Rolfing Movement will show you that your body is a healer, counselor, and friend. Or maybe you've been looking for a physical complement to an inner awakening. You've pounded the pillow, released tears of grief and rage, and finally resolved a painful past experience. You respond to life with new maturity until, unexpectedly, some situation triggers your old response. The earth is once again unsteady beneath your feet; with dismay, you find yourself reverting to old, outmoded behaviors. More emotional catharsis or mental analysis of the issue may not be what you need. The key to the completion of your transformation may lie within your physical structure.

Whatever your reason for being interested in your body, you'll benefit from becoming aware of gravity's impact on it. We're all playing the Gravity Game, whether we're aware of it or not. Gravity *always* wins. We can be winners too if we learn the rules of the game.

How to Use This Book

Balancing Your Body: A Self-help Approach to Rolfing Movement is organized as three parallel presentations. The first part of each chapter presents concepts and principles involved in your body's relationship to gravity, along with descriptions of "explorations" that will help you experience the principles for yourself. The explorations are simple movement patterns that establish gravity's freest neuromuscular pathways through your body.

The second part of each chapter tells the story of four people who just happen to be reading a book about gravity's influence on the body. You'll follow Bill, Margie, Pauline, and Fred as they explore the exercises in the book and share their questions, experiences, and insights. Though the characters in the story are fictional, their experiences are based on the structural problems and solutions of actual Rolfing Movement students. The narrative is meant to make the discussion of physical principles come alive and to provide examples of what might happen if you take this book to heart and really do the explorations.

Finally, interspersed within each chapter is a set of scripts for physical explorations. Since most of these are to be done lying down, you'll find them easier to follow if you have a partner read you the instructions or if you listen to an audiotape. You can purchase the companion audiocassette for *Balancing Your Body,* which contains a selection of these movement explorations read by the author, or you can make an audiotape for yourself. The effectiveness of the explorations depends on your being in a deep state of relaxation; therefore, many of the scripts are written in a hypnotic rhythm. The scripts include ellipses between key phrases to signal a pause when reading. Record or read the instructions in a calm, slow voice, leaving plenty of time between sentences to feel or do what's called for.

Though simple, the explorations are powerful and can evoke unexpected emotional responses. Chapter 9 offers guidelines for emotional self-help, and the appendix lists resources for professional assistance.

Think of this book as your Rolfing Movement coach. You may wish to read it straight through at first, skimming the scripts; this will give you a bird's-eye view of where you're headed. Even if you're reading it quickly for an overview, when the narrative directs you to sit in a certain way or move around the room, it's important to get up and do so *right then.* Subsequent discussion assumes that you've had the sensory and kinesthetic experiences suggested. The book will make much less sense if you read it in a sitting position only.

And promise yourself to go back and *do* the explorations. In order for the concepts to affect your body and your life, you have to give your physiology some new experiences. Plan on spending several days on each chapter's explorations. Changing physical habits takes a little time.

Because the experiences are cumulative, I suggest you do the explorations in the order in which they're presented. The depth of your experience of script 13 depends on your having thoroughly experienced script 3.

The explorations are just that, "explorations." They're not exercises you can benefit from by doing in a rote manner. They require your full attention and awareness. Their purpose is to uncover new internal sensations that you can use to redesign the way you move through your life. In most cases you need to go through an exploration only once or twice, enough to gain sensory experience of the concept being explored. The goal is not to continue practicing exercises, but to incorporate the concepts of support, fluidity, and congruence into your daily life. Scripts 5, 20–22, and 31 are designed for integrative experiences and can be used as ongoing review.

CHAPTER 1

BLUEPRINT FOR STRUCTURE

Here's a simple experiment to remind you of the way gravity works. Pick up a pencil or another small object lying at hand. Now drop it. Do this several times and watch the force of gravity in action. Feel what's happening to the pencil as if *you* were the pencil. Silly as it seems, if you do this you'll gain respect for the balancing act these bodies of ours are performing each time we take a step. We, of course, have more alternatives than a pencil with respect to gravity's pull. But the feat of vertical locomotion on two hinged stilts is something most of us take for granted.

The simplest model of stationary balance in the body is a stack of blocks. Suppose you wanted to build a human figure out of Lego blocks. You'd select blocks for feet, calves, thighs, pelvis, midriff, rib cage, neck, and head, and then you'd stack them up. You'd pick blocks of even lengths for the leg segments so your pelvis would be level, and you'd carefully align the torso segments to insure the head's safety on the top. Any block that might be misshapen or twisted or tilted out of line would be an opportunity for gravity to reduce your Lego figure to its generic parts. Luckily for us, our bodies' "blocks" are safely ensconced inside layers of skin and muscle; otherwise we too might end up as heaps on the floor.

Our bodies are amazingly malleable, able to accommodate all sorts of deformation and still continue functioning. When gravity

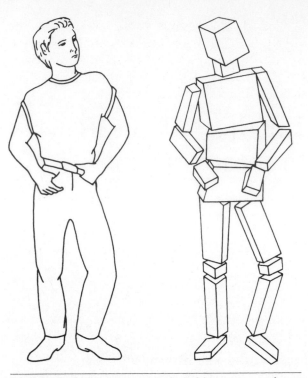

Figure 3: *This teenager's habit of bearing weight on his right leg and hip is likely to result in low back pain when he's older.*

tugs downward on our misaligned blocks, muscles in between those blocks contract to keep them in place. An imbalanced body, however it's bent, twisted, and compressed, glues itself together with tension in order to remain upright under stress. The result is a body that is tighter than necessary and that functions as if it were shorter and thicker than it really is. The mechanical definition of the word *stress* implies the resistance of elastic tissue to external forces. That's what we do—we resist gravity's pull by compacting ourselves, and in the process we reduce our ability to respond to stress with resilience and mobility.

Sound like a lecture to stand up straight? Not really. Our goal is balanced bodies in action. At the moment, we're just looking at how the blueprint for static structure affects movement.

At the simplest level, your body is like a stack of blocks: when the

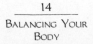

blocks are properly aligned, your body is stable and spacious, the tissue at once resilient and relaxed. When the blocks are crooked, the "plastic factor" in your body cements them together, distorting your shape and restricting your ability to move. Let's look at how the mysterious malleability of the human body works.

The Plastic Factor

All the parts of your body—bones, muscles, organs, blood vessels, and nerves—are surrounded by and intermeshed with a semi-elastic fibrous material called connective tissue or, to use its anatomical name, fascia. To help you visualize your fascia, picture an orange. The orange has skin around the outside of it, a membrane around its individual segments, and a thin film separating the tiny particles of fruit within each segment.

Imagine all these layers communicating with and affecting one another. That's how the fascia is interwoven within your body—the superficial fascia is an all-encompassing sheath just under your skin and is directly connected to the fascial sheaths around your individual muscles and internal organs, even to the membranes around cells. Fascia stretches like knitted fabric—if you snag your sweater on a nail, the whole garment is pulled out of shape.*

Combine this concept of interconnecting plasticity with the picture of the body as a stack of blocks: if one of the blocks is cockeyed, the fabric that interlaces them will pull on the other blocks as well. All the parts of your body intercommunicate through the fascia, with complex patterns of compensation resulting from any one incident of tension.

The main ingredient in connective tissue is the protein collagen. Collagen has the fascinating quality of being able to change in texture from something like gelatin to something more like glue or even leather, depending on how it's being used.

When a body block is askew, muscles in the surrounding area contract to hold the misaligned part in place. To feel what this is like, lift your right shoulder toward your right ear and hold it there

---

*The analogies to the orange and the snagged sweater are Dr. Rolf's. See *Rolfing: The Integration of Human Structures* for her inimitable discussion of fascia.

while you finish reading this paragraph. Doing this requires spending energy. To go on contracting your shoulder muscles indefinitely would waste a lot of energy. So your fascia comes to the rescue. When a body part, like a shoulder, is chronically out of alignment, the normally elastic tissue that surrounds and interpenetrates the muscles involved changes to a leathery consistency. Now tough and inelastic, it effectively fixes the shoulder in place. Your muscles become short and tight and stop being able to fully respond to your desire to relax them. Eventually the sheaths around adjoining muscles get bonded together, restricting the range of motion in the joint.

Scar tissue is an example of tough, inelastic connective tissue that forms around an injury when the body needs to repair and protect itself. Scar tissue restricts movement at the site of the injury. Structural imbalance is like an accumulation of mild injuries to which your body has responded by becoming tougher and less mobile all over.

Your Fascial Pattern Dictates How You Sit

Freeze. Don't move a muscle. More than likely, you're sitting in a position that is usual for you. Let's take a moment to look at the structural design of the way you sit.

Start by noticing the orientation of your pelvis. Are you settling more into one buttock than the other? Does one hip feel more compressed by the weight of your torso? Are you sitting forward on your thighs or back on your tailbone? Is one leg crossed over the other? Which way?

Now notice the orientation of your rib cage in relation to your pelvis. Is your rib cage closer to your pelvis in front or in back, on the right or left side? Where are the tips of your shoulders in relation to your chest? Is one shoulder higher than the other? more forward than the other? And your head: is one ear higher than the other? more forward?

Now reverse your sitting pattern—cross the other leg over, shift your weight to the other buttock, curve your spine in the other direction, raise your other shoulder, and adjust the tilt of your head. Make as exact a reverse replica of yourself as you can. How does it feel? If it feels somewhere between terrible and very strange, you're among the majority of people.

The first sitting position, the comfortable one, expresses your fascial pattern, your body's preferred way of orienting itself. Your fascia has accomodated to the pattern of compression and rotation in your body so that your slightly off-kilter sitting position feels secure. As you'll see later on, your fascial pattern dictates the way you usually stand and how you're likely to use your body in every move you make.

What About Exercise?

"What about it?" you ask. "Surely my poor alignment is just a matter of not enough exercise. If only I could find time to get to the gym. . . ."

One of the benefits of exercise is that the rhythmic contraction and relaxation of muscles acts like a pump to aid your heart in circulating blood through your body. When movement in an area of your body is restricted by thickened connective tissue, though, the pumping action of the muscles in that area is inhibited. This then restricts the flow of cleansing fluids and nutrients through the bloodstream. The misaligned area becomes a two-fold target: for injury because of its restricted flexibility and for disease because of congestion and the accumulation of body toxins. Thus, poor body alignment and the immobility it causes may conceivably lead to arthritis or other incapacities of the aging process.

Current research indicates that exercise will alleviate and even reverse some of the diseases of aging. Because so many people have been taking exercise seriously in the last few decades, the senior citizens of tomorrow should be a livelier group than our present-day elders. But exercise alone won't reverse the Gravity Game. In fact, without proper alignment you can actually reinforce your imbalanced habits with exercise.

If your blocks are out of alignment, you'll tend to work your body along the patterns of stress already embedded in your fascia. Let's say it's easier to bend your torso to the left than to the right. If you're not familiar with your structural pattern, you're likely to aggravate it by overstretching the side that moves easily, thus catering to your restriction. In strength building, you'll tend to

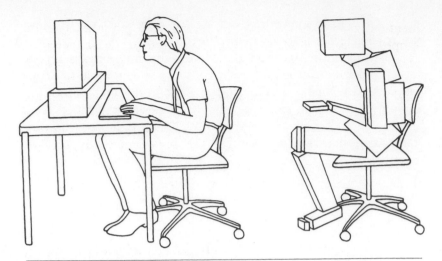

Figure 4: *A long day at an ill-fitting workstation restricts this man's breathing and sends him home with neck and shoulder tension.*

push yourself to the limit of your already stronger side. Imbalanced body usage of this sort leads to injury.

Changing Your Movement Habits

Repetitive use of your structure effectively molds your shape. It's easy to recognize the thickened neck and shoulders of a football player, the turned-out thighs of a ballerina, the bowlegs of a cowboy, or the hunched shoulders and forward-reaching head of a computer programmer. The nervous system tells the muscles what to do, and connective tissue accommodates. The neuromuscular system gets into a groove, recognizing a command and executing it over and over in the same way. In time, the shortened fascia dictates a path of least resistance for your movement. This is called a habit. Habits seem efficient because they're familiar. The premise of Rolfing Movement is that you can restore your structure to balance by changing the movement habits that perpetuate imbalance.

Not all movement habits are as easy to identify as the ones

mentioned. Let's say you fell down a ski slope ten years ago and limped for six months afterward. Even though you've forgotten about those months of discomfort, your fascia still bears a faint imprint of that limping pattern, just enough so that when you walk, you step slightly harder on the leg that wasn't hurt. There are lots of other reasons why you might prefer bearing more weight on your left leg. Maybe your dad's preference was to support himself on his right leg. To achieve rapport with him, you might have unconsciously mirrored his stance.

Fascia adapts to the way it is used, thickening and toughening along the tension lines of a particular stress. The orientation of the connective-tissue fibers reinforces the body so similar future pressures can be met. The fascial pattern becomes obsolete and limiting when the original stress ceases. Sometimes people identify with their fascial patterns to the extent that they unconsciously put themselves in situations that simulate the original pressure. For instance, a person who was browbeaten as a child adopts a defensive posture in relation to the world. His mature stance in life is hampered by attitudes of subservience or defiance. Over time, the attitude congeals into a fascial pattern that is a way of knowing who he is. The fascia is then a physical prison that fosters cycles of dysfunctional behaviors.

If the self-perpetuating spiral of imbalance and stress is allowed to continue, gravity wins the game. This outcome can be reversed through awareness, release, and the formation of new habits. Awareness comes first because you can't release an imbalance until you know it's there.

Sometimes the process of releasing these tensions evokes memory of the original stress. However, it's not always important to determine the source of a habit. What is important is the creation of new neuromuscular options so old habits can stop limiting you. Once tension is released, the body has to find a different orientation so the fascial webbing can readjust. This is done through conscious practice of new movement patterns. The movement re-education revises your internal sense of balance and ease. In time, the new balance becomes familiar and the new way of moving feels better than the old. New habits then provide physical support for improvements in self-image and behavior.

Getting Acquainted
with Your Structure

Script 1 helps you take the first step toward awareness of your structural patterns. For the walking evaluation, choose a room or corridor where you can go twenty paces without having to turn around. Walk purposefully, as if you were going across the room to open a window. Go back and forth until the pace and rhythm of your gait feels ordinary. Continue walking while your partner reads you script 1 or while you listen to the tape you made. Not all the questions will be applicable to everyone: pay attention to the ones that seem pertinent to you.

SCRIPT 1

EVALUATING YOUR STANDING AND WALKING PATTERNS

Start by standing comfortably in your stocking feet. Shift your body around until you are in a position that feels familiar, the way you would be standing, say, if you were waiting in line at a theater. Are you comfortable with your body weight settling more into one leg than the other? . . . Do your feet turn outward or inward? . . . Do your knees lock? . . . Are you leaning most of your weight on one hip? . . . Try settling your weight into your other hip and notice whether that feels as comfortable. Then assume the more familiar stance again.

Notice what you are doing with your arms. Are they crossed or placed akimbo on your hips? . . . Is the positioning of your arms a way of making your torso feel stable? . . . How does your rib cage line up with your pelvis? . . . Are your hips forward and chest depressed, . . . or are your buttocks thrust back and chest forward?

And how about your head? . . . Does it balance easily on top of your spine, . . . or is your neck tense from holding your head in place? . . . And your jaw, . . . does your chin jut forward or is it pulled in toward your throat?

Begin walking now, taking a minute to get into a familiar rhythm. Pay attention to the sound of your feet on the floor. Continue walking until you would recognize the sound on a tape recording. How hard or how lightly do your heels strike the floor? . . . Does one foot seem to come down more emphatically than the other? ... Does one leg take a longer stride than the other?

Notice how far your rib cage is from the ground as you walk. It is a distance you will sense kinesthetically, not something you need to measure with a yardstick or see in a mirror. Get a good feel for it. Does your chest seem far from the ground or close?

Consider that your body has an upper half and a lower half. Where is your sense of the demarcation line? ... at your hips? midriff? upper chest? It's not the same for everyone.

Stop walking for a moment and stand relaxed. If your walking were controlled by a motor inside your body, where would the motor be located? ... When you take your next step, from where arises your impulse to move, ... from the upper half of your body or the lower half?

Find the center of your chest, the general region of your heart. Where is your heart in relation to your knees and feet, ... in front of them or behind? ... Does it feel like your heart is reaching to impel you forward, ... or are your hips driving forward while your trunk lags behind? ... How about your head? Does it feel supported by your heart or does it stick out in front of your chest?

Just for fun, exaggerate the characteristics you've just noticed about your gait. Chances are the exaggeration feels familiar, something like the way you feel on a bad morning. Don't despair. Remember, your structure is plastic and its blueprint can change.

You have just completed a preliminary exploration of some of the characteristics of your structural blueprint. You will have opportunities to reevaluate and discover more about your standing and walking in succeeding chapters.

Take a few moments to make note of what you recognized about your body after listening to the script. Jot down your impressions so you'll have a record to refer back to as your body changes.

Be objective about what you observe, but not judgmental, cultivating a friendly attitude toward your structure as it is. No one responds to education by being browbeaten, least of all your own body. After all, your tensions and imbalances have resulted from your body's best efforts to keep you together under the stress of your life. Have respect for those old efforts as you seek to add alternative ways of being in your body.

In chapter 2 you're going to discover how your structure responds to the most basic movement of life—breathing. Awareness of your breathing pattern will help you experience firsthand how responsive your body really is. But first let's meet Bill, a member of our fictitious Gravity Gang. Bill is an ordinary, "thirtysomething" guy who stumbled into caring about his structure during his mid-life crisis.

The Gravity Gang

"Hey, Stringbean," teases Mike, "why don't you land on your brains next time?" Billy, victim of a growth spurt at age ten, rubs his bruised tailbone and picks up the accursed skateboard that trips him at every curb. He withdraws into a world of video games where play isn't painful. Landing in the street so many times has caused him not only to believe he's uncoordinated but also to slightly contract the muscles around his sore behind. Billy tucks his pelvis down and under even more in response to the spankings he sometimes receives from his dad.

As he grows, Billy's pelvis is in a poor position to support the length of his spine. To compensate for the imbalance in his torso, he acquires the habit of slumping and poking his head forward, which also helps him to reach the eye level of shorter comrades. Peering at video games makes this habit even more pronounced.

In high school, Bill's height makes him excel at basketball, and his social life takes a turn for the better. He's a bright student who goes to college and gets a good job, childhood difficulties behind him. But his slung-under hips and stooping shoulders portray a lack of confidence that doesn't match his real capabilities. In fact, he always looks a little abashed, as if somebody had just hooted, "Hey, Stringbean."

Bill is aware that his childhood wasn't the greatest, though he doesn't really think of himself as being emotionally scarred. The compression of his body tells another story. He has a few physical complaints—mostly neck tension and occasional headaches—that he alleviates by taking aspirin. It never occurs to him that the source of his distress might be the tension in the seat of his pants.

Bill's wife left him recently. It was rotten timing, the same week the company passed him over for promotion and the week of the NBA playoffs. Fortunately the Lakers won. But now Bill needs something else to boost his spirits, to help him feel stronger, more powerful. Maybe weight training. . . . But you can see it coming, with that spine and pelvis: a primetime weight-room casualty. And, in the Gravity Game, another round for gravity.

Bill has decided to ease into his fitness program gradually with a low-impact aerobics class. His blood hasn't circulated this much in years. The instructor, a cute woman in shiny blue tights, looks terrific doing the routines. Bill does his best to imitate her moves, but when he catches a glimpse of himself in the mirror, he has to laugh—baggy maroon gym pants, knobby knees pumping, arms flailing, panting like a dog. If this is the road to "shape," he has miles to go.

On the way to the locker room, Bill notices his posture in the mirror. No wonder Kay left him, he thinks. Who could love a slouchy looking guy like that? He prods his body into a remembered picture of good alignment—something about a plumb line passing through ear, shoulder, hip, and knee. There. That looks better. But the moment he takes a step, perfection vanishes.

Bill is determined to do something about his self-image. Browsing in the bookstore one day, he comes across a book that discusses the body as structure, as architecture that moves. This idea appeals to Bill. He remembers way back to his days in Sunday school and how Mrs. Edwards used to talk about the body being a temple. The book explains that his body is being rebuilt from moment to moment according to a kind of blueprint and that he can change his posture by relaxing. That sounds like a way to go.

A thorough type, Bill looks up the word *posture* in the dictionary. It means to put or place something, or strike a pose. No wonder posture has always felt like so much work. "If I can balance my structure by changing my old habits," he says to himself, "then I can create a new me." He pulls out his wallet and pays for the book. "It makes sense," he thinks. "You've got to change the blueprint if you don't want the same old design."

Bill isn't someone to do things halfway. He's taken up tennis for another means of exercise. By now he's learned a thing or two about his movement patterns, and he can adjust his structure while he practices his serves. Sometimes he has to stop and take a deep breath: those old habits don't give up without a fight. But Bill now knows that the minute he starts making an effort, he's installing an undesirable new tension. When the old clumsy feeling takes over, he packs up his racquet and calls it a day. Sometimes the hardest habit to curtail is the habit of trying too hard.

In time, Bill's attention to his structure pays off. His body begins to feel freer and lighter than it has in a long time, perhaps ever. For fleeting moments a new internal sensation takes over, and Bill feels like the man he wants to become. Something is happening outwardly too. Friends notice he's more assertive at work and seems to walk with more energy. The boss is wondering if he might have short-changed Bill in the past.

CHAPTER 2

EVERY BREATH
YOU TAKE

"How's it coming?" asks your boss. "Whew," you gasp, snatching the tearsheets from the printer and handing them over. You're panting as if you've just climbed a fourteen-thousand-foot peak. Racquetball three times a week takes care of your aerobic conditioning, so that's not the problem. Fact is, you've been concentrating so hard on getting that report done by noon that you've hardly taken a sip of coffee, let alone a deep breath.

Isn't it strange that we should need to stop what we're doing in order to breathe? The apparatus of life is designed to consume oxygen. Without breath there is no life, yet many of us spend long portions of our days breathing shallowly or not at all. Smokers solve the problem by inhaling tobacco—smoking gives them an excuse for a moment's pause, not just for a hit of nicotine, but for a few full breaths as well.

A power lifter compacts his trunk around the air he breathes in, making himself solid against the five-hundred-pound weight he's about to heft. Likewise, many of us try to stabilize our bodies by holding our breath as we shoulder our burdens. And though our burdens may sometimes seem to weigh five hundred pounds, restricting our breathing is not an effective means for handling them.

Efficient and full use of your breathing apparatus is your first defense against gravity's downward pressure. To understand how this works let's look at the apparatus of respiration—the lungs, the rib cage, and the diaphragm.

The Anatomy of Breathing

The diaphragm is a dome-shaped muscle that lies across your midriff, separating your chest from your abdomen. When the diaphragm contracts, it flattens and moves downward, creating negative space in the rib cage so air can rush into the lungs via suction. You feel a slight expansion in your abdomen as the diaphragm contracts.

The rib cage is more than just a bony fence that surrounds and protects the lungs. Tiny muscles crisscross the rib cage, causing it to operate like a cylindrical set of Venetian blinds. With each breath, individual ribs rotate ever so slightly as they move up and down. Other muscles expand the rib cage front to back and side to side. Optimally, all of these muscles help the diaphragm draw air into the lungs.

As you remember, all muscles are encased in and interconnected by the network of fascia that encompasses the entire body. As the muscles involved in breathing perform their pumping action, the fascial network responds. Your whole body participates in breathing, down to your baby toe. Once your structural awareness is tuned up, you'll be able to feel this.

There are several structural benefits to having the rib cage participate fully in your breathing. Movement of your rib cage raises the upper part of your torso away from the pelvis, leaving more room for your internal organs. When you slouch and hold your breath, your internal organs are squeezed between your diaphragm and the floor of your pelvis. They have difficulty functioning optimally under such conditions.

Another advantage to a mobile rib cage is that it promotes resilience in your spine. The tips of each pair of ribs attach to a corresponding vertebra, so when your ribs move, your spinal column lengthens. This movement eases tension in the back and restores the spine's ability to cushion your weight as you move about.

A third benefit of full-body breathing is that the increased dimension of your upper rib cage gives your neck and head a base upon which to rest. In a slumping posture, with your rib cage collapsed, your head lacks support and your neck must strain to hold your head up, inviting neck tension.

Singing teachers and athletic coaches often emphasize abdominal rather than full-body breathing. Psychotherapeutic practices based on the teachings of Wilhelm Reich also advocate abdominal breathing, as do most meditation schools. For activities that require such techniques, it's fine to continue them. Structurally balanced breathing is not considered a priority for achieving operatic, athletic, or spiritual satori. However, once you bring breath into the torso and your rib cage begins moving freely, you can evaluate for yourself whether or not the structural improvement is beneficial for your special avocation as well.

Breathing Evaluation

Lie down on a firm surface and breathe in your everyday manner. If you've been practicing a particular breathing method such as deep abdominal breathing or timing your breath to a numerical count, put that practice aside for now. Valuable as such methods are, they may sometimes mask your real breathing pattern, which is what we want to get acquainted with right now. So simply breathe as though you were settling down for a short nap.

Observe your breathing for the next ten cycles. Notice the rhythm of your inhalation and exhalation. Which part takes longer? Which part feels easier? Which do you enjoy most? Is there a pause or hesitation at any point in your breath cycle? Where is that?

What parts of your body seem to be moving as you breathe. abdomen? lower chest? upper chest? shoulders? You may be amazed to feel how little your rib cage moves.

Now take a fuller, deeper breath. You'll sense more movement in your rib cage this time; you'll likely also notice more effort. Memorize the sensation of your effort—on a scale of one to ten, how hard is it for you to take a full breath at this moment?

Next, stand up and get acquainted with your breathing in an upright position. Notice where you feel movement within your body as you breathe. Gauge the effort you needed to take a deep breath.

In this chapter, you're going to practice two types of breathing. We'll call the first type *fascial breathing*. Its purpose is to draw your attention to the movement that occurs in the rest of your body as you breathe. Once that awareness is available to you, we'll go on to *structural breathing*, which will help you improve the structural balance in your rib cage.

The value of attending to breathing has been known for centuries. Sufi, Yoga, and Taoist disciplines all encourage various manipulations of the breath that lead to altered states of consciousness by changing the oxygen content of the blood. Hypnosis also emphasizes breathing. In the exercises that follow, you'll be paying attention to your ordinary breathing pattern. Avoid deep or regulated breathing, or anything that requires effort. The scripts will help you become more aware of your breathing than you usually are.

For these exercises you'll need to lie on your back on a firm but comfortable surface such as a carpeted floor or an exercise mat. Place a cushion under your knees to reduce strain in your lower back. If your head is tilted way back or if your throat feels constricted in this position, place a small pillow or folded towel under your head.

Your Breathing Cycle

Script 2 focuses your awareness on the rhythm of your breathing. Your body's demand for oxygen changes from moment to moment. Some breaths may be long and full, others short and shallow. The important thing is that your exhalation is complete. Many people avoid or rush this part of the breathing cycle. Exhalation is controlled by the part of the nervous system that is also in charge of relaxing muscle tone. This means that if you don't exhale completely, you are sabotaging your body's natural inclination to relax. The respiratory pause is the completion of the exhalation. It causes the CO_2 level of the blood to signal your nervous system for the next intake of oxygen. If the pause is completed, the ensuing inbreath feels effortless and full because it is triggered by your body's automatic physiological demand for more air.

◆

SCRIPT 2

EXPLORING YOUR RESPIRATORY PAUSE

Lie comfortably on the floor with your knees on a cushion and your neck supported on a folded towel that feels comfortable. Let your body settle into the support of the floor. Once you feel comfortable you can start becoming aware of the rhythm of your breathing. Notice how long it takes for the air to come in, ... and how long it takes for the air to go out.... And one way may seem easier, ... coming in, .. or going out. ... And one way feels more pleasurable.... And there's a moment at the top of your inbreath, ... when your lungs send your brain the message that they are full. Then your breath releases and the air flows out. And at the end of your exhalation, there's a pause, ... while your body decides to breathe in once more. You find that this pause can take a short time, ... or a long time. Each time you breathe out you discover how long the pause wants to be. This moment in time is the center of your breath, ... a moment of rest. You let yourself feel peaceful during the pause, ... during that vacation in the middle of your breathing, ... a vacation right in the middle of your life.

And take a moment, before you return to reading, to appreciate your breath.... When you are ready, let your eyes open and gently come to sitting.

Fascial Breathing

The third script asks you to become aware of the movement of your breathing in different parts of your body. Let's say you're sensing the movement of your breath in your forearm. When you do this, it's not an actual flow of air that causes the sensation in your forearm. What's happening is that by focusing your attention on your arm as you breathe, you're able to feel the fascial movement that is always occurring there, whether you're aware of it or not. Try that now. Can you feel the movement of your breath in your forearm? If not, try imagining what it might be like to feel that movement. Picture the fascial layers in your arm gently spreading out as you inhale.

Script 3 begins by directing your awareness to the movement of your breathing through your left side. Before going on to the right side, it's useful to pause and notice how each leg feels. You'll probably sense a difference between them, as if your left leg had more weight, dimension, energy, or aliveness. Then repeat script 3 for your right side.

Once you're breathing through both legs, stop again to notice how they feel. They'll tend to seem more of a matched pair. It's possible, however, that they may still feel quite different, as though one leg were heavier or larger or warmer than the other. They may seem to be made out of different qualities of clay or even to have contrasting personalities. This feeling is due to a difference in your *body image* of your legs.

Body Image

Your body image is your neurological sense of yourself—how your brain senses your body.* It develops through your experience and use of your body. For example, a person who has lost a lot of weight may retain a "fat" body image. She developed a certain way of moving to carry those extra eighty pounds, and though the pounds are gone, she still moves in the same way. Scales and dress size tell one story, but her movement says she is still overweight.

Bill, our friend from chapter 1, retained an awkward, adolescent body image well into his adult life. Having grown so rapidly—twelve inches in one year—he had trouble matching the small-boy sense of himself with the manly stature he suddenly acquired. The upper and lower parts of his body felt disconnected. His legs seemed thick and rubbery, while his chest and arms felt thin and the middle of his body seemed vacant. Bill's impulse to try weight lifting reflected his wish to change his body image into one that would be strong, connected, and competent.

Your body image, distinct from your self-image, is usually an unconscious factor in the way you carry yourself. You may live in your body as if you are fat or awkward without being aware of it. Once conscious, those images can be transformed into images of balance, grace, and integration. Changing your body image changes the blueprint for your structure. The first step is to become aware of and appreciate your body image as it is now.

If your legs do feel significantly different from each other after you listen to script 3, it's an indication of structural imbalance in your support system. Remember your habitual standing posture? More than likely, you're comfortable bearing more of your weight

---

*See Jean Houston, *The Possible Human,* Chapter 1: Awakening the Body, for a beautiful presentation of the concept of body image.

on the side that now feels larger or more dense. You'll learn some ways to even out this type of imbalance in chapter 8. For now, just notice this aspect of your body image without judgment or concern.

The rest of script 3 extends the sensation of fascial breathing through your torso, arms, and head. Your whole body breathes together. Fascial breathing develops your sense of relationship between any part of your body and any other part. You could feel your right hip and left shoulder breathing together, or you could feel your eyes breathing with the soles of your feet.

The fascial breathing script assists you in exploring your body image. It's like taking an internal reconnaissance flight. Your breath is the vehicle in which you ride around inside your own skin. The terrain of your internal landscape can be very diverse. One place within your body may seem dense or hard and difficult for your breath to move through. Another place may feel empty or mushy or prickly. The images you receive could include colors, shapes, temperatures, even sound.

Don't worry if you're not able to feel all the sensations as they're suggested in the script. Your awareness will develop and deepen as you practice. Just imagine that you feel them. In this way, you can give your perceptions a jump start.

SCRIPT 3

FASCIAL BREATHING EXPLORATION

Lie on your back with a cushion under your knees and a folded towel under your head if desired. Start becoming aware of the rhythm of your breathing. . . . Letting the rhythm of your breathing, . . . with its little pause, . . . remain in the background of your awareness, you notice now the movement of your diaphragm, . . . as you breathe in and out. . . . And you may notice that this movement causes a slight pressure in your pelvis. You sense this pressure in your left hip, as it comes, . . . and goes. . . . You feel it like the gentle rocking of a boat, resting in a quiet harbor.

And the rocking sensation fills your left buttock. You follow that sensation down into your left thigh, . . . as your thigh softly pulsates to the rhythm of your breathing. Now your knee seems to be pulsing, as if there were a little lung inside your knee, and the lung fills up as you breathe in, . . . and empties as you breathe out. . . . And noticing how the back of your calf gently rests against the floor, . . . your calf relaxes, . . . as the movement of your breath, . . . travels down through your leg, . . . into your left ankle. And your breath smoothly ebbs and flows, . . . through your left hip, . . . and left leg, . . . down to the sole of your foot. Your whole left side seems to be getting longer, . . . each time you breathe in, . . . and settling deeper into the floor.

As you continue breathing, you notice the way your left leg feels, . . . and the way your right leg feels. And one side may seem very different from the other.

And sensing the movement of your breath once more in your diaphragm, . . . you follow the sensation down into your pelvis, . . . and you feel a gentle rocking in your right hip.

Repeat from second paragraph, changing "left" to "right."

With your breath moving through both of your legs, you can now begin to feel an echo of that movement through your arms. . . . You may notice how your breathing causes a slight expansion in your left shoulder joint. And the space between your upper arm and your shoulder might seem like the space between two boats moored side by side in a harbor. . . . And the gentle undulation of the tide seems to travel down through your arm, . . . through your elbow, . . . forearm, . . . and wrist. It might seem as though the bones of your arm are floating there, inside your skin.

And now you begin to spread the sensation of your breath, moving like a tide across to the right side of your body. Spending all the time you need, you feel the gentle undulation of your breathing in your right shoulder, . . . through your right arm, . . . elbow, . . . and wrist.

And you find it easy to feel this pleasant, undulating movement through your arms, . . . and legs, . . . at the same time. As you do this, you find that your spine is just naturally included, so there's a gentle breathing motion up and down your spine as you inhale, . . . and exhale. Your spine seems to be settling ever more deeply into the mat. And now you might even be feeling the gentle ebb and flow of your breath inside your head, . . . between your ears, . . . behind your eyes, . . . and under your tongue.

BALANCING YOUR
BODY

Spend a few more moments with this pleasant sensation, . . . imagining that every cell in your body is breathing. . . . Your whole body is renewed with fresh energy. . . . When you are ready to return to reading, let your eyes open and come to sitting.

◆

Structural Breathing

Once your body awareness has intensified through fascial breathing, you may begin noticing freer movement in your rib cage. Script 4 helps you release the movement of your rib cage even more.

If you're like most people, your body image of your rib cage comprises your chest—the front half of your ribs only. Chances are you've never thought about your rib cage having side and back dimensions also.

Script 4 directs your awareness to new possibilities for movement within your rib cage and to the interrelationship of structures in your torso. Think of your torso as a vertical tube. Across the tube lie three main horizontal dividers. The topmost is the dome-shaped ceiling of your upper rib cage, the bottom is the floor of your pelvis, and the middle is your diaphragm muscle. These structures are like drumheads, and your breath reverberates between them.

In the beginning, you may find yourself inhaling deeply as you attempt to feel your ribs moving in unused dimensions. Gradually assume your normal breathing depth and rhythm, and let the visualization process instill the new pattern. Mental intention has greater effect than physical effort in transforming body/mind habits.

Developing a new breathing pattern will change your experience of your whole body. Toward the end of the script, you'll be asked to attach some descriptive words to this experience. You may sense an uncommon warmth in your body, a feeling of transparency or of greater depth or dimension. You might feel as though a rainbow were swirling through your body, or you might "hear" your body humming a tune. Whatever your experience, describe it specifically to yourself.

The next instruction will be to undo the new sensation. This is an important learning step. Notice what adjustments you make to undo the new sensation. What specific tensions do you replace?

Then practice re-creating the new sensation. Without going through the entire script again, simply replace the heavy or tense state with the more expansive one you achieved by following the earlier instructions. This undo/re-do process helps you plant the new neuro-muscular information into your body, like seeds in a garden. As you practice the new patterns, the seeds will bear fruit.

Focusing on your breath is a powerful experience. Even though the purpose of these explorations is structural awareness rather than meditation, the deep relaxation and focus will alter your state of consciousness. Always spend a few moments stretching and "coming back to reality" after practicing the exercises in this book.

SCRIPT 4

STRUCTURAL BREATHING AWARENESS

Lying comfortably on your back, become aware of the rhythm of your breathing. . . . Let your breathing rhythm and your fascial movement continue in the background of your awareness. With your palms resting lightly somewhere on your torso, . . . move your attention to your first three ribs, the ones just beneath your collarbone. These ribs form concentric circles inside the top of your chest. As you breathe, the circles expand outward in all directions. . . . As they expand to the front, you can feel your collarbone rise slightly. . . . As the circles expand sideways, you can feel more space across your upper chest, between your armpits. . . . And when you relax your upper spine, you can let the circles expand toward the back, . . . inviting your breath into the space between your shoulder blades. . . . The circles expand in all directions. . . . And when you exhale, . . . your body softens, . . . and a sense of release deepens within you.

Now your shoulder blades are just drifting, riding on the motion of your rib cage. You may even notice your upper ribs sliding smoothly across the inside surface of your shoulder blades. Take all the time you need to let the rhythm of your breathing smooth away the tension around your shoulders. . . .

And now you can let your awareness move down inside your chest,

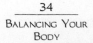

as if you could travel down inside to the location of your heart. And you spend some time there gazing up at the dome-shaped ceiling of your ribs above you .... It's like the ceiling of a cathedral or the high vault of a mosque. You watch the dome gently pulsating as your breath flows in and out. Above, you sense your throat relaxing, ... and your neck and head resting on the gentle rhythm of your breath.

Moving your attention down to your midriff, ... you can feel the motion of your diaphragm, a gentle expansion in your upper abdomen. And you notice the sides of your midriff, how your ribs expand sideways, ... and your rib cage widens as you inhale. And you can feel your lower ribs in back, ... floating on the tide of your breath. Or perhaps you can see them gently opening and closing, ... like Venetian blinds.

Now you notice how your diaphragm and upper rib cage move together. As your diaphragm descends, your upper ribs expand in all directions, ... like an umbrella unfolding. And the umbrella relaxes as you breathe out.

Below your waist, you begin to feel the resonance of your breathing in your belly, ... in your lower abdomen, ... in the floor of your pelvis. You can feel your breath moving across the back of your pelvis, ... down along your sacrum to your tailbone. And the floor of your pelvis echoes the motion of your diaphragm as you breathe in and out.

As you breathe, you notice how the top of your rib cage, ... and your diaphragm, ... and the floor of your pelvis, ... all move together. Your whole body expands and lengthens with each inbreath, ... and softens with each exhale. You feel the potential for deep peace.

Turn your attention now to the overall sensation in your body at this moment. How would you characterize this sensation? If you could see it, what would it look like? ... If you could hear it, how would it sound? ... If you could touch it, what would be its temperature, texture, shape?

Now, knowing that you can re-create this sensation whenever you wish, find out what it's like to stop feeling it. Undo the feeling, carefully noticing how you achieve this. Where do you tense up again? Where do you close yourself down?

Then, remembering the feeling you had before, bring it back, ... color, texture, shape, sound, ... your breath moving all through your body once again. Carefully notice how you do this. Your personal imagery is your surest path to freer breathing.

Now, begin returning to an ordinary state of awareness. Let your eyes open. Look around at objects in the room. Notice their shapes and colors. Feel the texture of the carpet under your body. Notice sounds in the world outside. Find a comfortable way to sit up, bringing the new sensations with you.

◆

Emotional Responses

Some readers may experience unexpected surges of emotion while practicing these or other Gravity Game exercises. You may experience moments of sadness, anger, fear, relief, or gratitude. You don't need to feel this way for the structural work to be effective, but if you do, you may wonder why.

Emotions, like body image, affect the blueprint of your structure. To understand why emotional feelings might arise while learning to improve your breathing pattern, let's consider why we stop breathing under stress.

For most of us, there has been a time when we felt threatened and, for one reason or another, were not able to respond by "flight or fight." Instead, during those instant freeze-frames, we metaphorically turned ourselves into stone. The physical response is similar whether the stimulus is dire or mild—there's a rush of hormones, increased heartbeat, a sharp intake of breath, a sudden muscular cringing. Like a rabbit at the scent of a predator, our bodies become utterly still—for that moment, breathing stops.

To become so still as to be invisible is a strong, primitive survival response. In time, we learn that holding our breath and tightening our muscles is an effective way to feel safe under any circumstance—this response effectively shields us from abusive elders, taunting schoolmates, loneliness, and rejection. The habit may become so ingrained that it shields us from our success and joy as well as from our pain. The tension has become incorporated into the blueprint for structure.

The part of the nervous system responsible for your survival remains primitive despite the sophistication you acquire as you mature. You may be vice president of a major corporation, with all the latest technology at your fingertips, but in a time of crisis—a corporate merger, for instance—your ancient survival mechanism gears up for disaster. You may behave with apparent control, even managing well under the stress, but there's a tight stillness inside, a shallowness of breath that hearkens back to the way you learned to survive in childhood.

What happens when you focus on your breathing is that you start letting go of the habit of stillness. You discover that bracing yourself is only one of many possible responses to stress. As the movement of your breath makes your body feel fuller and more flexible, the part of your body image concerned with breathing begins to shift from a feeling of threatened survival to competence and ability to cope. When the shield of stillness is laid aside, it may reveal the feelings and emotions hidden behind it. Memories of times when the shield was needed may surface.

Some people may perceive such feelings physically, while others may have visual images as if they were experiencing a waking dream. Some may hear sounds or voices. Let yourself experience these fragments of feeling or memory, knowing that they are being released because your body is relaxing chronic tension. You might see those feelings or memories being played out as if you were watching them on an imaginary movie screen in front of you.

As the emotions reach resolution, your body will feel as though a "stuck place" has been freed or a weight has been lifted. Generally, a release of emotion that comes through releasing physical tension is brief and is followed by a feeling of relief. However, you may wish to seek professional help should emotions arise that do not easily resolve. Various approaches to body/mind therapy are discussed in chapter 9, and a list of referral sources for practitioners is given in the appendix.

Special Breathing Problems

Some people, especially those with pronounced lower-back curvatures, have difficulty feeling motion of the lower-back ribs. Pronounced lower-back curvature presents as a back that is very tight and rigid, and a spine that grooves deeply at the waist. If this is true for you, you may find it helpful at first to work with the breathing scripts while lying on your stomach. Place a cushion under your abdomen to support your lower back. Chapter 4 will help you understand your back tension, and the movement pattern in scripts 12 and 13 (pages 73 and 76) will help you relax your lower back.

If you have a history of asthma or other respiratory illness, pay particular attention to the movement of your breastbone. The asthmatic breathing pattern draws the lower end of the breastbone inward on inhalation. This pattern may persist, distorting the rib cage, long after the respiratory disorder has ceased.

Lying on your back, rest your hand across your solar plexus. Relax the muscles of your upper abdomen—feel them softening under your hand. Focus your attention on your breastbone, and notice it rising and falling as you breathe in and out. Imagine the bottom tip of your breastbone rising toward the ceiling as you inhale. Don't force it to rise—just *picture* the movement as vividly as you can. Changing an asthmatic breathing pattern may take some time, but the potential freedom in your chest is well worth your patience.

Breath Awareness
Changes Your Walking

Before you go on to the next paragraph, please review script 1, the walking evaluation (page 20).

Now, sit on a firm chair with a seat high enough that your hip joints are slightly above your knees. Support for sitting will be discussed in greater detail in chapter 3. For now, sit toward the edge of the seat without leaning against the back. Bring your pelvis upright so you can feel your sitting bones beneath your trunk. Distribute your weight so your trunk is resting into your pelvic basin and your legs are supported by your feet. With this broad base of support, your spine can be at ease without inclining. Now, in this position, review script 4 on structural breathing (page 34).

Once you can feel the full dimension of your breathing in the sitting position, stand up and bring the fullness with you. Feel the dimension of your breath in your pelvis, midriff, and rib cage—front, side, and back. Then begin walking back and forth as you did in chapter 1.

Compared to your previous walking, how loud do your footsteps now sound? Is your rib cage the same distance from the floor or slightly farther away?

If the breathing explorations have been effective, your walking will feel lighter and easier now. You may feel more connection between your upper and lower halves. Your footfalls will sound quieter. You may even feel taller. This is because releasing your rib cage relaxes and elongates your spine, restoring its ability to cushion your weight as you move. As your structural awareness develops during the ensuing lessons, your sense of lightness and ease will increase. As you become accustomed to it, this new balance will begin to feel like the "real" you.

Walking is a matter of falling and catching yourself. You can do this gracefully and efficiently or in an effortful, haphazard manner. It's inefficient for you to lift or push your weight forward each time you take a step—you're using more energy than you need to. When your spine elongates as a result of correct breathing, your center of gravity is high, just above your navel. Since your body is already lifted, you don't have to raise it for each step. That's why you feel and sound lighter.

Breath Awareness
Changes Your Appearance

That old admonition to change your posture by pulling your shoulders back never worked because it did nothing to change the foundation on which your shoulders rested. When your rib cage is able to expand in three dimensions, your torso lengthens, your shoulders broaden automatically, and your slouch disappears. And breathing with your rib cage also has a beneficial effect on the "battle of the bulge." Take a look at your profile in a mirror: what happens to your abdomen when you're breathing in this new way? A slumped torso puts such downward pressure on your abdomen that it has no choice but to protrude.

You can't cheat though. Just lifting your chest and holding it there won't do the job. Forcing yourself into a new pattern will inhibit your freedom of movement as much as or more than your old one. Pretty soon you'll be tired and crabby, and your habitual breathing pattern will reassert itself. In order to really change the structure of your torso, you must take the time to change your internal blueprint for breathing.

Review the breathing explorations enough times for the new pattern to be comfortable before you go on to the next chapters. Set aside time to practice breathing just as you would schedule time to learn any new skill. Remember that in addition to opening new neuromuscular pathways, you may also be revising a deeply ingrained pattern of defense. Notice any part of your body where the movement of your breath is difficult to feel. Since this may be an indication of both structural imbalance and emotional shielding, give that part plenty of attention. Even five minutes of practice a day will keep the new sensations fresh in your awareness. Success in changing your habits depends initially on conscious intention. Gradually, your nervous system will prefer the new breathing pattern, and you'll find yourself doing it automatically.

Applying Breath Awareness to Daily Living

To begin incorporating full-body breathing into your daily routine, try the following process. Lie comfortably on your exercise mat. Imagine yourself performing some simple task such as doing dishes or filling the car with gasoline. Picture yourself doing this as if you were watching a scene in a play. See the clothes you're wearing, feel the movements of your body, hear the clatter of the dishes, feel the soapy water on your hands, and notice the pressure of your feet against the ground. Notice also the way you're breathing as you imagine the scene. Feel any constraint across your chest or abdomen, any tension in your neck and shoulders.

Then forget the scene, and spend some moments evoking your sensation of full-body breathing. Feel the gentle expansion of your ribs, the three dimensions of your torso, the connectedness of your arms and legs. Enjoy the ease as your body settles into the exhalation. Once this feels comfortable, conjure up your scene again. This time, split your attention so you can continue the fuller breathing pattern while you watch yourself at work. Do you sense a change of energy in the way you're performing the task?

Apart from the change in your breathing, what's the difference between the two ways of using your body? Find words to describe it. Switch back and forth from one way to the other until you're aware of specific differences in the way your body feels. Next time you actually do the dishes or fill the gas tank, design the task to include your fuller sense of breathing and the different quality of movement.

Try this process with several simple, familiar activities so you'll have some specific times in your day that are repatterned with full-body breathing. In this way you can have fun weaving your new physical awarenesses into your life and find yourself feeling better too.

The Gravity Gang

Bill has an interesting experience with the breathing awareness scripts. The first time through he can't feel much of anything. Then he decides to focus on his respiratory pause—maybe that's more important than he'd supposed. The funny thing is, he suddenly finds himself feeling anxious, even a tiny bit scared. It's as if lengthening the pause might make him miss out on taking his next breath. It's an odd feeling, almost like drowning, though he never had any trouble swimming that he can remember.

Bill finds it strange to be lying comfortably in the cozy atmosphere of his home, feeling afraid of not being able to breathe. It makes no sense at all to his logical mind. Curious, he watches himself experiencing this strange yet somehow familiar sensation. Bill's study of meditation practices some years back makes it easy for him to separate himself from his experience.

Watching now, Bill has a vague impression of himself as a little boy, long ago, hiding from something. He sees himself shudder, frown, and then, as if a weight were being removed from his chest, take a full, deep breath and exhale slowly.

Bill's anxiety gradually dwindles, and he feels increasingly comfortable taking longer pauses between breaths. The pause begins to seem like a vacation from the activity of breathing. The more he allows himself to take this rest, the deeper and easier his breathing becomes. It feels peaceful.

Suddenly Bill feels his knees doing something unusual. They seem to be getting bigger and smaller, as if they too are breathing. Looking down, he can't see anything strange happening to his legs. What do you know, he thinks, fascial movement!

This is a fine moment for Bill, whose wife always complained that he wasn't subtle enough. As Bill continues exploring his breathing, he finds that, for him, the respiratory pause is the key. All the other changes of movement and awareness flow naturally from that. But if he forgets the pause, everything else feels artificial.

Bill lies on the floor, feeling more relaxed than he has since his honeymoon. He wonders what Kay would think. She had disliked his meditation practice, complaining that he was distancing himself from her. But body awareness seems like something she'd like. Maybe it would even help her PMS. . . . Maybe they could talk things over. "One step at a time," an inner voice counsels him. "First you've got to learn to stand on your own two feet."

When Bill stands up, his body feels smooth, his joints well lubricated. He walks around the house, does the dishes, and then takes a shower, humming a tune, high on his own breathing. Out of the shower, he stands in front of the mirror. What a disappointment: he still looks like a slouch. Kay would scoff. As he pictures her reaction, his chest tightens and his breathing grows shallow.

His thoughts shift. The feeling of expansion in his chest was so dramatic a while ago. Where is it now? Bill wonders. The Gravity Game seems so logical, there must be something he's missing. Then it hits him: but of course—it's *gravity* that is missing. "Gravity was supporting my whole body when I was lying down," he mutters. "I haven't learned how to support that open feeling when I'm standing." He gives himself a shake, takes a deep breath, and climbs into bed. There must be more to this standing up than meets the eye.

CHAPTER 3

HOW TO THROW YOUR WEIGHT AROUND

Support for Your Intentions

"Walking is a matter of falling and catching yourself." You may have skimmed over that sentence in the last chapter without making sense of it. Well, for most people it *doesn't* make much sense. Most people don't fall forward as they walk—the majority thrust their feet forward and pull their trunks along behind. But watch a toddler catapult across a room—the child wants to see what that bright yellow object is. She focuses on her goal and hurls her whole body toward it. In a moment your antique teapot is a collection of shards. Adults add finesse to their execution of intention. They also often add shyness, fear, defensiveness, embarrassment, insincerity, guilt, or any number of other counterintentions to their actions.

Our counterintentions are usually not conscious and often are not even derived from present-time experience. Our friend Bill was hardworking, smart, and capable, and yet a part of him didn't seem to want to get ahead. There was something self-effacing in his carriage that said, "No, Stringbean, you'll never make it." When Bill relearned what the toddler knows instinctively—to get his weight behind his intentions—his whole life improved: on the tennis court, in the office, and at home.

Margie, the personnel director at the company where Bill works, has been selected to participate in a team-building pilot project. The program includes a week of guided mountaineering with a wilderness education school. The climax of the week is a peak ascent to fourteen thousand feet. Although she's in good shape from weight training and running, Margie is terrified of heights. "Keep your weight over your feet," calls the climbing instructor. Margie's shoulders are cinched up to her neck, her chest is hunched, and she's barely breathing. As she gingerly reaches her left boot to the next boulder, she leans her shoulders to the right. Fear counter-weights her intention to get to the top.

Any skier will testify that your legs will slide out from under you on the slope unless your body weight is centered. The minute the top half of your body is incongruent with what your legs are doing, you're bound for a tumble. Yet even if you're an expert skier or mountaineer, the kinesthetic concept of "weight over your feet" is something you can still learn more about. Humans have an interesting capacity to master skills in an area of great interest and challenge, while letting the basics erode. Have you ever noticed how a ballerina walks in her street shoes? Isn't that swanlike neck a strange match for those duckling feet? Most everyone's body image has an incongruous part or two.

Let's find out how well your structure supports your weight and how well your gait expresses your intention to get ahead. We'll start by examining your ordinary standing posture.

Balance of Front and Back

Standing comfortably in your stocking feet, notice how your weight falls through the soles of your feet. You'll feel this as pressure against the carpet. Is there more pressure on your heels or on the balls of your feet? To evaluate this, rock your body back slightly until you feel your weight pressing squarely down on your heels. Notice how the muscles across the fronts of your ankles, thighs, and abdomen must contract to keep you from falling backward. Now lean forward hinging at your ankles so your weight settles over the balls of your feet. In this position, you'll be gripping your toes, your arches, your calves, and your buttocks. Sway very slowly back and forward again, noticing how each position affects the relationship of tension in your legs, abdomen, back, and shoulders.

Imagine that your body can be divided into a front half and a back half—like the two sides of a sandwich. Pay attention to your body image as you support yourself with the front half of your body, leaning on the balls of your feet. Then settle back on your heels, and sense the difference in that position. Most likely, your body image will seem thick and dense in the supporting half, vague or empty in the passive half.

Keep rocking back and forth, gradually reducing the sway until you recognize a central zone where you feel supported by both halves of your body. Standing in this zone, your weight is evenly distributed between the balls of your feet and your heels. You bear your weight through the "palms of your feet," just as you would through the palms of your hands if you were doing a handstand. We'll refine this awareness later on, but for now, visualize your footprints evenly indenting wet sand. Notice that the muscles of your feet, ankles, and knees are hardly working at all. The truer the balance, the less tension you'll feel.

Now shake your body out a bit and resume your original stance. If your weight settles naturally into your heels, your heelprint will be deeper in wet sand. If you bear your weight forward, the toes will be deeper.

Working with a partner, here's another way to evaluate your support system. Have your partner stand on a chair behind you so that, with his hands on the tops of your shoulders, he can gently press straight down through your body, toward the floor. Have him do this while you stand in your usual manner. Notice where you feel the added stress in your body. Does it make your back start to buckle? Do you feel strain in your shoulders or possibly in your neck?

Now have him press down on your shoulders with your weight evenly distributed over your feet. Your partner should imagine that he is pushing straight down through the middle layer of your body, between the front and back halves of the "sandwich." This time you should feel the stress as a generalized pressure that goes down through your torso and legs to the palms of your feet. In this case, the added pressure is shared by all the parts of your structure; no one specific part is overburdened.

Pushing and Reaching*

If you watch people walking, you'll notice that many push themselves forward with the lower half of the body, while others reach forward with their arms and chests, legs pumping to keep up. In either case, the top and bottom halves of the body reflect different intentions, and the body's motion is not congruent. Most people literally don't "have it together." How does your movement express your intention to get where you're going?

In a few minutes we'll evaluate your usual gait, but first, let's sample some of the ways other people locomote. We'll do this theatrically by improvising some exaggerated, imbalanced gaits. By purposefully being off-balance, you develop a need for balance and a sense of how balance really feels. Have fun with these explorations, but remember that imbalance does cause strain. Don't get so creative that you hurt yourself.

First, walk with your feet kicking forward from your knees. Let your heels dig in a little with each step. Exaggerate: let your chest sink down, and push hard into the ground with your feet. Feel your energy in the lower part of your body—pelvis, thighs, and feet. Except for your head, which juts forward, your upper body lags behind your legs. Try to intuit the feelings or attitudes of someone who would walk this way. Who is this character?

Try another. This time, instead of pushing with your legs and pelvis, reach forward with your arms and chest. Your vitality is now located in your upper body, and your legs are like distant cousins that you barely know. As your chest thrusts forward, your pelvis stays behind and your hips swivel a bit. You've just created a sway back. What's happening to your head and shoulders? You'll either feel tension between your shoulder blades from holding your shoulders back, or tension in your neck from retracting your chin. Whenever one body part is out of balance, another body part

---

*I am indebted to Rolfer Hubert Godard, who pointed out the difference between "push" people and "reach" people at the 1990 Rolf Institute International Conference. His observations could easily fill another book.

will also be out of balance, the pieces being held together with tension. What kind of character walks like this?

One more: tuck your tail under and lead with your pubic bone. This guarantees that you'll slouch and waddle. Let your heels drag along the floor as if you were wearing your grandfather's slippers. Notice how stiff and rigid your spine becomes, how hard it is to breathe. Where do you feel your energy this time—upper or lower body? Another minute of this and you'll feel old age setting in.

Now walk in your usual way. Whew! What a relief. Contrast your familiar pattern with the exaggerated movements you just enacted. Do you sense more vitality in the top or bottom half of your body? Do you push forward with your legs and pelvis as you walk or reach with your arms and chest? Do you spend more time on the leg that strides ahead or on the one that pushes off from behind? Where is the center of your chest—your heart area—in relation to your legs? Are you ahead of yourself or behind? Are you more aware of the front or the back? Appreciate how much your awareness has grown since you first evaluated your gait in chapter 1.

Now walk across the room with all of your attention on the front half of your body. Then shift your attention and continue walking, paying attention to the back of your head, back of your spine, backs of your legs. Notice how shifting your attention changes the quality of your movement. Which way feels more familiar?

Exaggerate your familiar walking pattern. Who is *this* character? What mood does this characterization express?

The scripts in this chapter develop your ability to sense physical support for your intention, to feel your body congruent in its action. All parts move together, front and back, top and bottom, combining the energies of reaching and pushing.

The Back of Your Body Image

Many of us bear our weight over our heels, supporting ourselves with excessive tension in the back half of the body. This is one reason why it's more difficult to feel the movement of breathing through the back half—the excess tension masks sensation. Another reason is that we tend to present ourselves to life frontally—our backs don't seem very important to us, so they're hard to feel unless they hurt.

Script 5 is an exploration of the back half of your body image. In this experience, you'll first focus your attention on the movement of your breath throughout the front half of your body; the sensation of fascial movement is generally more accessible in front. Then you'll gradually blend the responsive feeling into your back half, releasing the tension there. Avoid forcing your breath into your back—effort will sabotage the relaxation you hope to achieve. Instead, imagine that your back has already become more pliable and responsive—all you have to do is feel it.

◆

SCRIPT 5

EXPLORING YOUR BACK HALF

Lie on your floor or exercise mat with a cushion under your knees and a small pad under your neck if that feels comfortable. Let your palms rest on your midriff.

You're breathing in an ordinary way, letting the air easily come and go as your body requires it, . . . allowing for a slight pause at the end of each exhalation. The front half of your torso rises toward the ceiling each time you inhale, . . . your abdomen gently expands, . . . your chest and collarbone float on the tide of your breath. Your throat softens, . . . your jaw softens, . . . the muscles inside your mouth, . . . under your tongue, . . . and behind your eyes . . . soften.

And as your breath flows easily down from your head, . . . down within your trunk, . . . through your legs, . . . to your feet, . . . your breath plays through the front half of your body like a soft ripple in a quiet tide pool. . . . And you find your own words to describe the sensation. Maybe the front of your body is filled with light or color. Maybe it is soft, . . . or hard, . . . warm, . . . or cool. Maybe it pulsates, . . . undulates, . . . hums.

And now you move your attention to the back half of your body, . . . noticing the different sensations there. You appreciate the texture of your back: its color, . . . temperature, . . . and density. You appreciate your back for its hard work in supporting you for so long,

. . . and let your back feel what it's like to not work so hard. . . .

Now you begin to marry the sensations in your front and back halves, letting the colors and textures blend: letting what is hard grow softer, . . . letting what is weak borrow firmness from the other side, . . . taking all the time you need.

With your palms resting on your solar plexus, your attention moves to the ribs in back, just above your waist, . . . and breathing easily, those ribs begin expanding just a little. And you notice your breath moving easily into the back half of your rib cage, . . . carrying relaxing sensations with it.

Now, moving your palms to rest across your lower abdomen, your attention moves to your pelvis, . . . and letting your buttocks muscles relax, . . . you can imagine the dense back wall of your pelvis softening, . . . responding to the flow of your breath. . . . As your pelvis settles more comfortably into the mat, you can follow the movement of your breath along the inside surface of your sacrum. . . . And your abdomen feels soft, . . . as it relaxes fully into your pelvic basin.

Now your attention wanders upward through the back half of your torso to your upper spine. Laying your palms across your upper chest, you feel the rise and fall of your breathing there, . . . and when you soften the area between your shoulder blades, . . . your whole body can surrender to gravity.

And your breath moves through the bowl-shaped curve at the back of your head. . . . Your cranium seems soft now, . . . as it widens and deepens in rhythm with your breathing.

Still savoring the pauses in your breathing, . . . focus your attention on the back half of your body. . . . Your body seems to be resting more deeply into the floor. And the sensation of weight and relaxation in the back half of your body streams down through the backs of your thighs, . . . backs of your knees, . . . calves, . . . ankles. The back half of your body is now completely at rest against the mat, . . . and your front half softens into the back, . . . and gravity supports you.

Now slowly undo the sensation of support, carefully noticing the specific places in your body that become more compact, more closed, more tense. And then, remembering your breathing, re-create the sensation of support.

When you are ready to resume your usual state of awareness, allow your eyes to open. Notice your surroundings. You can sustain the

*sensation of support by gently rolling to one side and pushing yourself
to sitting.*

Your Core of Support

Remember when your partner pushed down through the middle layer of your body from above? This is the core of your structural support—when your weight is balanced over the palms of your feet. When free of tension, your core is fluid, resilient, and responsive to your body's ever-changing demand for balance. It's possible, however, that your core is not free but is instead braced against past or projected painful experiences. This deep and vulnerable area of your body may be associated with feelings you're not consciously aware of.

Script 6 evokes the sensations and imagery of your central core. This middle layer might be very thin, like a layer of Greek pastry; it might seem like a round tube or a brightly colored ribbon. It may range in texture from water to steel. Take all the time you need to evoke your core imagery. Take time also to explore any emotional associations. If you need help, refer to chapter 9 for approaches to emotional processing. When the emotions resolve, you'll feel an increased sensation of fluidity in your core.

SCRIPT 6

EXPLORING THE CORE

And now you are going to shine a light on the core of your body, starting in the region of your solar plexus. Lying on your floor or exercise mat, with your attention on your midriff area, explore the interface between the front and back halves, . . . noticing how your breath moves between them. And this middle layer may be very thin, like a thread, . . . or it may be a vast open area. It is unique to you.

Now follow the interior space slowly and sensitively down through your abdomen, . . . into your pelvis, . . . and take time to breathe and explore the core of your pelvis, . . . the place between the front and the back. Let yourself appreciate the precious internal sensations there.

And now you find a corridor down through your right thigh, . . . knee, . . . calf, . . . and ankle, . . . to the sole of your foot, . . . and through your left thigh, . . . knee, . . . leg, . . . ankle, . . . and foot. And as you breathe through your core, you can feel a response in the palms of your feet, . . . and your legs seem to lengthen a little each time you inhale, . . . and as you exhale, a soft feeling permeates your whole body.

Now you travel back up through the corridors of your legs, to your pelvis, . . . abdomen, . . . upper chest, . . . throat, . . . and head. And you find your own words to describe your images and sensations of the middle layer of your body. . . .

And then undo that sensation, erasing the awareness of your core, . . . noticing the difference in feeling. And then, using your breath, restore your core awareness.

Now you imagine that the surface you're lying on could be upended and you magically find yourself in a standing position. You can allow your weight to be supported through the core of your body, . . . resting into the palms of your feet. You imagine the slight pressure of your breath through the soles of your feet, as if your breath were connecting you to the earth.

Now begin returning to an ordinary state of awareness. Gently let your eyes open. Look around at objects in the room and feel the texture of the surface under your body. Listen to familiar sounds.

◆

Standing Up with Core Support

Script 7 helps you maintain the feeling of central support as you actually get up from the floor. You'll be rolling your body upward from kneeling to standing, moving very slowly. Pretend you're experiencing your evolution from four-footedness to erect human posture. An important clue to finding core support is having your foundation in the palms of your feet.

Right now, as an experiment, lie down and then get up from the floor in the way you normally would, noticing the qualities of your movement. By contrast, the following exploration will show you how much smoother, lighter, and more grounded you are when supported by your core.

People who tend to initiate movement by thrusting forward with the lower body will feel taller when they discover core support. Those who initiate movement by reaching forward with the upper body tend to feel shorter or more compact—finding core support helps them settle deeper into the earth. The core helps integrate front and back, upper and lower, reaching and pushing.

◆

<u>SCRIPT 7</u>

ROLLING UP TO STANDING

Lying on your floor or exercise mat and remembering the sensation of support within your core, lazily roll your body onto one side, letting your knees bend and your legs curl in. Let your body give in to the floor as you pause for a moment on your side.... Then use your arms to push yourself to a sitting position. Feel yourself moving through your middle layer as you rise from lying to sitting. . . . Repeat this motion several times, allowing your nervous system to incorporate the sensation of supported motion. Notice how the front and back halves of your body cooperate in this movement. Now lie down again and get up as you would normally do it, noticing the difference.

Move once more from lying to sitting in a supported way, and then roll over onto your hands and knees. Tuck your toes under and shift your body weight onto your feet, letting your upper body hang loosely forward, head dangling. Pause and remind yourself to breathe. Slowly straighten your knees, balancing your weight over the palms of your feet, halfway between the balls and heels. . . . Let your knees stay relaxed in a soft bend as you continue upward. . . . Slowly roll your sacrum downward until your pelvis is level, still centering your weight over the palms of your feet. . . . Now with your arms, head, and shoulders still hanging forward, unfold your abdomen and midriff, breathing through the core of your body.... And as the core of your chest region gradually settles over your insteps, . . . your shoulder blades automatically slide toward your back. . . . And when your neck unfolds, . . . your head finds balance on top.

Take stock of your body right now. Does it feel taller, . . . fuller, . . . more mobile, . . . more relaxed? Does this way of standing affect your breathing?

For contrast, stretch and move about for a moment and let go of the awarenesses you've just achieved. Think of a specific situation in the course of your day when you would find yourself standing and waiting for something. Assume your usual stance. It is probably a little different from the new way of standing.

Now, slowly weave the sensation of core support into that specific situation. Bring in just enough of the new sensation to feel comfortable. In that specific time and place, you can feel a little more supported through the palms of your feet. . . . You can sense the dimension of your body, . . . and the movement of your breath through your core.

◆

Walking with Core Support

Script 8 helps you develop core support in walking. Though the feeling of resting into the core may still feel new or somewhat vulnerable, you're probably beginning to find it more readily. The core is mobile—it flows and pulsates with life. Bodies are never static, no matter how dignified, disciplined, or immobile we are.

Once you've completed script 8, you'll be able to understand the statement "Walking is a matter of falling and catching yourself." The impetus for moving forward is a concerted shift of weight in your trunk—head, chest, and pelvis together. Mind, heart, and gut feelings become united in intention; the feet and legs support that intention.

Margie learned this—the hard way—on a mountaintop. "Put your hands in your pockets," called Pete, the climbing instructor. "Trust your feet, Margie." As Margie inched her way across the boulders, her arms flailed at her sides as if groping for a handrail. Then she gingerly thrust her hands into her pockets and, in doing so, broke the pattern of counterintention in her upper body. Instantly the granite seemed steadier under her boots.

One foot after another, Margie followed Pete, imitating the way his feet contacted the rock. She tried to set her foot down in exactly the same spot, with the same confidence. When she remembered to breathe, she could almost enjoy the climb. Suddenly, as the group halted at the crest of the ridge, her trance was broken. Hands on her hips, knees barely quivering now, Margie looked out to appreciate the majesty of the Sierras.

Margie's scattered weight nearly sabotaged her intention to reach the peak. What you're learning in this next exploration is subtler and more precise than just putting your hands in your pockets, but the principle is the same: to let your legs support your intention.

◆

SCRIPT 8

STANDING AND WALKING

Remember your own descriptive words for the sensation of central support in your body. Allowing those words to guide you, walk across the room at an easy pace. Let your feet relax, so you can step into a soft, flexible foot. Your heel strikes the ground first with each step, but instead of landing there, your body's weight rolls forward through your instep and over the ball of your foot. With each footfall your weight drops through center into the palms of your feet.

Notice that your whole torso can move forward at the same time, front and back halves both guided by the core. Your legs, instead of leading you, are simply accompanying you. Notice the smooth articulation of the balls of your feet and your ankle joints. The top and bottom of your body feel connected to each other, so going forward seems to happen all at once.

How does this way of walking feel? Still unfamiliar and unusual, perhaps, but what else? smooth? more connected? more secure?

Stop a moment to shake your body out, and then resume walking in your habitual pattern. Gradually blend in some of the new sensations, keeping what you need of your familiar walking pattern and adding a comfortable amount of the new.

◆

In what ways is your walking different as a result of listening to scripts 5 through 8? What's the difference in your overall movement quality, the use of your energy, your mood? Play back and forth between your usual style of walking and the new. Keep what you like of the old way, and weave some of the new qualities into it. Find just the right blend.

Set aside five minutes once or twice each day to experiment with walking. Let this be a focused, contemplative time, separate from the rest of your daily routine. Notice any place where your body feels as though it's resisting the new pattern of support. This would indicate an area where you could spend more time releasing tension through the breathing processes.

Have an appreciative attitude toward any tensions that resist your new gait. The old habits have been holding you together, successfully, for a long time. It may take a little while for your body to understand that the new ways of support will be just as reliable as the old.

Tripod Support for Sitting

The last exploration in this chapter deals with supporting yourself as you sit. You'll need a bench or chair with a firm seat, high enough so that your hip joints are on a slightly higher plane than your knees. It should be low enough to let your feet feel firmly planted on the floor. If your chair isn't adjustable, use telephone books—under your feet if you're short or under your buttocks if you're tall.

Sit so you can feel your two sitting bones under you. Then locate your pubic bone, the midpoint at the front of your pelvis. If you could look down through your body from above, you'd see that these three points make a triangle. This triangle outlines the floor of your pelvis. The curving sides and back of your pelvic basin rise up from this triangular space.

Sitting with your pelvis centered in this triangle, your pelvic basin is level. Let your weight settle through your middle layer into your pelvis. Your knees are forward and your heels are directly beneath your knees. Feel the chair supporting your torso's weight through your pelvic basin and the earth supporting your legs through your feet. This tripod created by your two feet and your pelvis makes a very stable base for sitting, providing three points of support. Since the base of the spine, the sacrum, is free to adjust to your shifting weight as you turn in your seat, the rest of your spine is given mobility as well.

For contrast, sit in your usual manner. If you're like most people, you roll your pelvis back, so your weight rests on your tailbone and your abdomen caves in. You'll have little or no sensation of support from your feet. Compared to tripod support, this doesn't feel very grounded, or very balanced, or even very easy. Imagine how crowded your internal organs must be. How can they digest your lunch properly when they are compressed like this? And with your sacrum so anchored, responsiveness is diminished all the way up to your head.

A common mistake in correcting a slouched sitting position is to go too far the other way, sitting forward on the thighs, and hyperextending the lower spine. Strangely enough, although your body is leaning forward in this posture, you still feel little support from your legs and feet. This is because you have shortened the muscles at your groin, retracting your legs into your pelvis. Your energy is concentrated in the upper part of your body and your legs feel "cut off."

Have your partner push down on your shoulders from above as you sit in your usual position, and note any resulting strain in your lower back. Then, sitting with balanced tripod support, have him push down again. You'll feel pressure on your buttocks but no strain at any one point in your back.

Test both positions for ease and fullness of breathing. Which way supports the mobility of your rib cage in all dimensions?

Script 9 helps you develop a comfortable way to sit by moving back and forth between two extremes. As you alternate between a collapsed posture and a rigid upright, you'll find a place of balance and support somewhere in between. The extremely slow pace of this exploration lets you distinguish subtle variations in your internal sensation of support.

As you experiment with "tripod" sitting, you'll recognize that support is a "zone" rather than just one spot. "Sitting still" is a misconception from the past. Sitting is an activity, not stillness.

SCRIPT 9

EXPLORING THE SITTING ZONE

Sit on your chair with your pelvis centered over the triangular space between your pubic bone and sitting bones. Let your weight rest through your pelvic floor. With your knees in front of you, put your heels just under your knees. Sensing the movement of your breathing through your legs, . . . you can feel a minute pressure through the soles of your feet as you inhale. Notice the movement of your breath in your pelvis, in the front, . . . and in the back. . . . And follow your breathing upward through your core, from the floor of your pelvis, . . . up through your belly, . . . through your midriff, . . . and through your rib cage, . . . the flow of your breath expanding and releasing your whole body. . . . Relaxing your throat, . . . and jaw, . . . you can even feel the motion of your breathing in your head.

Gradually now, let your pelvis roll back and your trunk sink down into a collapsed posture. Notice that your legs are no longer helping to support you, that you are sitting behind the triangle of your pelvic floor, and that your breath can no longer move freely through your body.

Continuing to breathe comfortably, . . . and moving at the pace of a plant growing, begin rolling your hips forward through the triangle at the base of your pelvis. At each instant of this long journey, you can notice changes in your whole body, . . . the way your weight flows like a thick liquid, . . . very slowly down through your thighs, . . . into your feet. Still breathing comfortably, . . . your chest rides upward, . . . regaining its fullness, . . . your midriff unfolds smoothly, . . . and as you recover your core support, your neck and head find balance on top of your torso.

Now you continue rolling your pelvis forward, far forward toward the apex of the triangle. Now you notice that your legs have lost their easy, comfortable feeling, . . . and your spine feels like a steel beam, . . . no longer responsive to the movement of your breath.

Still breathing, . . . and moving very slowly, now let your pelvis roll back into the center of your pelvic floor, . . . and let your trunk settle into the spacious basin of your pelvis. Your legs feel supportive once again, . . . and your feet remember their contact with the earth. As the back half of your body relaxes, . . . you can sense your breath circulating

freely through all parts of your body. And the sturdy tripod base made
by your pelvis and feet, . . . feels like home.

And now, letting your body drift ever so slightly forward, . . . back,
. . . and to each side, . . . you can sense the perimeter of your sitting
zone, . . . and appreciate the generous way that your pelvis and legs
support you.

◆

Applying Tripod
Support to Daily Sitting

With your awareness of ideal support for sitting, you're likely
to find that the chairs you normally sit in no longer feel adequate
to the task. Chairs that have a bucket or depression, or that are too
soft, practically force you into a collapsed posture. Add a cushion
to fill in the depression or demand a firmer chair.

Adjustments to your work environment may be necessary. If
you find that you need to raise your seat, you may need to raise
your working surface as well. If you're working at a terminal,
adjust the height of the keyboard so your upper arms hang down
in line with your torso, elbows at ninety degrees and wrists flat.
The top of your screen should be at eye level.

If your feet dangle and there's no way to lower your chair, find
some way to raise the floor—a footstool or stack of books will do.
Though coworkers may snicker at your improvised ergonomics,
you'll have the last laugh when your back pain disappears and
theirs gets worse.

Spend the next few minutes exploring some of the basic
movements of working at a desk or table. Start the exploration in
your old sitting posture. Reach your arm across the desk to pick
something up from the far side. Notice how you're using your
body. If you're like most people, your pelvis stays behind on the
chair and you reach forward from your waist. You have little or
no support for the reaching action from your feet and legs. Since
your body is going in two opposing directions—back in the pelvis
and forward in the arms—your movement and intention are incongruent. Once you've picked up the object, your lower back has

to strain to return you to your original position.

Now sit in the new way, over your tripod. Remind yourself to breathe. To reach your arm forward, start by rocking your trunk forward from your sitting bones. As you pivot forward toward the apex of your pelvic floor triangle, some of your weight travels down your legs into your feet. Your waist, chest, and arms fall forward naturally, without effort. Because you use the momentum of your whole trunk to initiate the reaching action of your arm, completing the gesture feels light and easy.

To return to upright sitting, push your weight from your feet back into the pelvic triangle. Your upper body resumes its upright position without effort, motivated from below.

Improvise with this congruent way of using your body in the sitting position. If you reach for something to your right, reposition your foot a little to that side and take more weight on your right foot. Having finished your reaching action, push back with your right foot to re-center yourself.

If you have a sedentary job, you'll find it beneficial to envision and repattern several specific tasks that you perform every day while sitting at your workstation. Try one now—something simple like opening your mail. Sitting in your usual way, imagine yourself doing this activity. Imagine every detail: the feel of your clothing against your skin, the weight of the objects you're handling, the sounds you hear, the shapes and colors of your surroundings.

Observe yourself doing the task as if you were watching a video. Notice how your body is being supported. Notice your breathing and the quality of your movements.

Turning off the video, shift around in your seat until you feel tripod support. Watch a second video of the activity from this base. Describe to yourself the differences between the two versions. Review both videos a few times, so that when you perform this task again at work, you'll find yourself doing it with better support.

Under stress, we almost always revert to our familiar patterns, the old standby tensions that have seen us through many a rush job. Spend some time reprogramming an imaginary rush job.

Gradually, your body will begin to prefer the ease of being supported, and you'll find yourself less fatigued at the end of the day. This is predicated on having your chair and desk at the proper height for your body. Do whatever is needed to make your environment fit your body. To make your body fit the environment is an insult to your humanity as well as to your structure.

Dimension

For most of this chapter we've been considering the way your body can be supported from below—by your feet in standing and walking and your pelvis in sitting. But we've been working all along with the third aspect of support as well—dimension, the fullness of your body image.

Picture a basketball. The ball is supported only briefly by the point on its surface that strikes the court. What keeps it from collapsing between bounces is its internal pressure. In the case of the ball, this pressure is constant until the ball springs a leak. The body's internal pressure is a lot more complex and fluctuating than a basketball's. Speaking metaphorically, the ball, if it had awareness, would know itself on all sides. That's how it manages to spin around its center and land anywhere on its surface. Balancing your awareness of front, side, and back develops your sense of your body's three-dimensionality and helps you sense your center. Having awareness of your back and sides as well as your front makes you feel bigger, more substantial and stable, more "all there."

Be aware of your body's dimension as you repattern a familiar activity. Notice places in your structure where you tend to limit the space for your breath by hardening your body as you perform the task. Divide your attention between the action and your internal space. By breathing into the restricted area, softening and releasing any rigid places, you increase dimensional support for the action.

Rubbernecking

One way to refine your structural awareness is to watch other people moving. Visit a crowded mall or beachfront promenade where you can peoplewatch without being rude. Intuit the tension that goes along with the imbalanced structures you see. Notice the people who thrust themselves forward with their legs kicking their support in front of them, heels noisily digging in, upper bodies leaning back. Others tilt forward as if there were a phantom hand between their shoulder blades shoving them from behind. Still others bounce from their toes as if they were being led by the nose. Are their intentions supported by their structures? You'll begin to see how inept most people are at contending with gravity, and you'll gain compassion for their untutored attempts to play the Gravity Game.

The Gravity Gang

When Margie gets down off the mountain, she resolves to make some changes in her life. A self-confident and capable person, she is surprised to discover her fear of heights. Confronting this fear helps her realize that there are hidden stresses back home at sea level that she isn't coping with. But having climbed the mountain peak, she now knows she can climb her internal mountain if she commits herself to it wholeheartedly.

This is on her mind one day when Bill starts bragging about his tennis game—it seems he's been reading a book about "gravity awareness," and it's improving his game and his life. Just like Bill, thinks Margie. Ever since Kay left, he's been a full-blown mid-life crisis case. Every week he has fresh news about "human potential." But there is something different about Bill lately, Margie begins to realize. He's more outgoing, more self-assured. Even his voice sounds different—more . . . more what? His voice is more resonant: that's it "May I borrow that book?" Margie asks.

As Margie becomes more conscious of her body image, she discovers something interesting about her posture. As a young girl, her breasts had developed earlier than those of her peers, and she had been subjected to merciless teasing from the neighborhood boys. Though not particularly buxom now, she discovers a tension in her chest, a "pulling-in" feeling—it's like a shield. Out of curiosity, she exaggerates the shield.

As she walks back and forth across her living room, noticing how her legs push forward and her chest hangs back, she starts thinking about the street where she lived as a child. She's walking home from school, hearing those taunts. She stops, shuddering as if to shake off the unpleasant memory. Then she glances at herself in the hall mirror. There's a roundness to her shoulders—a shortened, even dumpy, appearance. She's beginning to look like her mother. She lies down on a throw rug near the fireplace.

As Margie explores the sensations of breathing in different parts of her body, she finds that her front half has a texture like Styrofoam, somewhat spongy and brittle, while her back half seems hard and sturdy like wood—except for those steel reinforcements in her lower back and across the tops of her shoulders. Margie is strong—she'd had to be. Her childhood had been a challenge. Her parents were always fighting and the little girl had been the peacemaker.

Margie had turned her survival instinct into a drive to get to the top of her profession. Her hard work paid off in terms of material success, but lately Margie has been reaching for something else, something she can't quite define.

At first, Margie has trouble imagining that her breath can cause motion in the back half of her body. Then she pictures air passing in between the cells of the wood. The wood somehow turns into a living tree, and then the tree's growth reverses backward in time until it becomes a tender green sapling. It is a gentle spring day long ago. Margie is walking through a forest with a little girl who is also herself. She is holding her own hand and explaining something to her younger self. The boys' mean words and laughter fade into the distance behind them.

"I must have dozed off," she muses. Now it seems to Margie as though the inside of her body is soaking in a warm bubble bath. The steel and wood and Styrofoam have all melted together and turned into . . . she squirms around and giggles . . . silly putty. "What a trip," she mutters.

"What in the world are you doing?" asks Pauline. She's noticed her roommate lying on the floor every evening for the past week. It's time for an explanation.

Pauline listens with interest as Margie does her best to explain "body image" and "core support" and "intention." "I don't really understand it myself yet," she says, "but you should see Bill. He's jacked his desk up on bricks and gotten himself a really tall chair. He sits up there like a king, telling everybody he's supporting his structure. It seems weird, but I'm telling you, the guy is . . . ," Margie searches for the right word, "blossoming."

"Blossoming! Bill?" asks Pauline, incredulous. "How exactly?"

"For one thing, he cracks jokes. He has a sense of humor. Kay used to tell me he was funny but I could never see it. He seemed like such a computer drone."

"Yeah, I remember meeting him at your Christmas party. He seemed like such a bore. Say, I wonder if this book could help me with my singing. You say it's supposed to improve your breathing, right?"

"Uh-huh. Maybe it would affect your voice production. Why not give it a try?" Margie asks. "Then we could work together. It would be fun."

Pauline catches on to the Gravity Game right away, and soon she and Margie find themselves engaged in almost nightly conferences about their growing awareness. Pauline is particularly impressed with the concept of body dimension. Years of vocal training have taught her a very frontal presentation of herself. "I feel like a movie set," she admits one day, "all color and light in the front and nothing but stiff scaffolding behind." But when she tries to fill out the dimensions of her body image and allow her back to feel softer, she runs into some internal resistance—her concept of what is "petite."

"How can you complain about feeling more relaxed?" Margie asks with amazement.

"I like feeling relaxed," Pauline says, "and it sure relieves that constant tension in my back, but . . ."

"But what?"

"It makes me feel fat."

"Look. Let's try an experiment," Margie suggests. "Do what you need to do to make your body feel as petite as you'd like."

"Okay."

"So how does that feel?"

"It feels thin . . . ," Pauline replies "and compressed, and tight—I can hardly breathe."

"All right. Now, let yourself spread way out inside. Just for now, occupy all of your internal space. Breathe into the full depth of your body."

"That's a lot more comfortable—and feels a lot bigger."

"Okay, Paulie, be truthful with yourself. How different are your external contours right now compared to when you made yourself feel thin?"

Pauline is quiet as she explores the two possibilities. After a while her face flushes and she sighs. "Not much," she shrugs.

Pauline is a friend of Margie's younger sister. Fresh out of college with a music degree, she hasn't yet found her niche in the city. She knows one thing, though: she hates waitressing. One evening she comes home with some new insights about her situation. "I was thinking about 'intention,'" she tells Margie, as the two sit down to dinner. "My real intention is to become a singer, not a waitress!"

"I thought you took that café job because the hours give you time for practice and lessons," Margie comments.

"Right." Pauline picks up a spoon and taps it on the table for emphasis. "So today I gave myself a lecture. I decided I might just as well pay attention to the way I use my body while I wait on customers. What's the difference if I'm on a stage or at the café? I'm in the same body!"

"So you might as well support yourself while you're waiting tables?"

"Got it. Centers of my feet, breathing, back dimension—the whole bit. And three things happened. One is that I'm a lot less tired tonight than usual."

"And the others?"

"Well, feeling three-dimensional out in the world feels—I don't know how to explain it. It feels sort of vulnerable, like it's easier to be flat—just a front."

"As if it's not safe to have all of yourself so available?"

"Yes."

"I noticed that too," Margie nods. "At first I could only let myself feel that fullness when I was alone. It seemed like a dimension of myself that I haven't felt for a long time—maybe since I was a little kid. I'm getting more used to it now, though. What was your other experience?"

"It happened during my singing practice. I was experimenting with dimension today, feeling the depth of my body. You know, appreciating the fullness rather than trying to be petite. Then I started thinking about my base of support and wondering about my feet." Pauline stands up to demonstrate. "See, we're supposed to stand with our feet close together, like this. But if I put one foot just a tiny bit ahead of the other, less than an inch even, I feel more stable. It seems to give my base of support more depth. So my voice gets better support." Pauline moves toward the door.

"Aren't you going to let me hear?" Margie calls after her. Pauline is shy about performing and Margie wonders what she'll reply.

"Maybe later," Pauline answers. "Let me tell you one more thing and then I've got to run." She's already halfway down the hall.

"What?"

"I figured out why singers get so fat," she calls from her bedroom. "I think they put on weight to make up for not being properly supported. It's a way of feeling grounded."

"Where are you off to?" Margie follows her down the hall.

"I've got a date with Fred."

"That cute guy with the sports car—not bad. What does he do?"

"A bit of everything, it seems: a stint in the army, manager of a fitness center. Now he's a sales rep for a sportswear company. Before that . . . oh, I shouldn't tell you." Pauline blushes.

"What?"

"Promise you won't let on that you know."

"I promise. Now, spice up my life."

"Well, he worked in a nightclub—as a go-go dancer."

"You're kidding!"

"Don't let those glasses fool you. The man has a great body, and he can really move. Now don't forget . . ."

"Well, at least I can *look,* can't I?"

"Okay." Pauline laughs. "But remember, I got there first!"

CHAPTER 4

THE PELVIS CONNECTION

Relay Station for Congruent Motion

Martial artists find the source of their power in the abdomen, about an inch below the navel. They call this spot the *hara*. This is the fighter's center of gravity. With knees bent and legs apart in a wide sparring stance, the muscles of thighs, buttocks, and trunk tighten around the hara, the source of all potential energy. Kicks and punches explode from a rock-hard core, but the center itself remains immobile. Such bodies are efficient and beautiful fighting machines.

Winning the Gravity Game requires a different type of power in the pelvis than that sought by martial artists. The fighter's hardened core provides support for sudden, forceful movements; our daily activities, on the other hand, don't usually require such force and speed. To move through daily life with ease, the core of the pelvis needs to be fluid and flexible—it should feel open, so the breath moves freely through it. The center of gravity can then shift higher or lower in response to changing situations.

Fred is a man on the move. A black belt in Tae Kwon Do, Fred is also proficient at scuba, skiing, and basketball. He's successful at his work: as a sales representative for a line of outdoorwear, he won a new car last year for being his company's top salesperson nationwide. Lately, though, he's been having some back pain—ever since a twenty-mile forced march at Army Reserve camp last spring. Sure, they'd had to carry a lot of heavy gear, but Fred's fitness program always prepared him for such rigors before. Now he notices that a day on the road visiting customers takes a toll on his lower back. He can stretch it out at the gym later, but it's annoying to feel like he has to pamper himself.

Trudging twenty hot miles with a heavy pack put a different set of stresses on Fred's body than two hours sparring in a clean *dojo*. Four hours behind the wheel of a car is another workout altogether. The pelvic tension that grants Fred those spectacular spinning jump-kicks works to his disadvantage in his daily life. Fred needs to learn how to release the tension in his pelvis when he's not practicing karate, so subtle impulses can be freely communicated between his legs, pelvis, and spine. The athleticism that has won him such fine muscle tone has made him too taut at his center. Fred is beginning to be constrained by his own strength.

Pauline has begun to relax the tension in her pelvis by letting go of her belief that tightening her abdomen makes her look slimmer. Tension in the abdomen is a common habit among women who think they're too plump. By squeezing in around the waistline, they force their abdominal contents down into a hard little pouch. This action is usually combined with a tucking of the sitting bones in an attempt to minimize the contours of the buttocks. Such girdlelike tension reduces freedom of motion in the hips. The restricted mobility impedes metabolism and may actually cause excess tissue to collect right where it is not wanted.

The pelvis is a relay station where the impulses to reach with the upper body and to push with the legs can be integrated into congruent forward motion of the whole body. Most people's pelvises lack the core mobility needed for this integration to take place.

The design of the pelvis is similar to a rock climber's sling or the harness on a small child's swing set. The back strap of the pelvic harness is formed of sturdy bone, while the front is enclosed only by muscle, allowing for freedom of forward motion. The hip joints correspond to the harness's leg openings. You can also visualize the pelvis as an internal saddle. Sitting with tripod support, imagine your weight settling into an old-fashioned, high-backed saddle. Your pubic bone is the pommel. You can remain supported by this saddle even when you stand and walk. When not restrained by inappropriate muscular tension, the pelvis operates as a combination sling and saddle, responsive to the actions of both spine and legs.

The explorations in this chapter develop the sensation of appropriate motion in the hip joints and lower spine, increasing the capacity for responsiveness in the pelvis and congruent motion of the whole body.

Evaluating Your Hip Motion

Walk across the room as you've done in previous explorations, this time with your attention on your pelvis. Does your pelvis feel attached to your legs or more connected to your upper body? Where do you feel the swinging sensation of your legs—at your thighs, in your hip joints, or higher up within your trunk?

Be aware of the center of your pelvis, the area behind and below your navel. Can you feel movement reverberating through that area as you walk? Or does it feel more like there's a brick in your belly, a still place that you have to swing your legs around?

Notice what your hips are doing. Some people will feel lateral (side-to-side) displacement of the hips with each step as their body weight settles into first one hip joint and then the other. This pattern is common in women.

Men tend to displace their weight laterally by shifting their upper bodies from side to side. They sway from the shoulders down, rather than from the waist down. A third common walking pattern is a swiveling of the pelvis around the lower spine, a gait made famous by Marilyn Monroe.

All three of these patterns make limited use of the rotational capability of the hip joint. Its ball-and-socket structure allows the leg a wide range of motion, but the most efficient action in forward locomotion is for the thigh to swing down and forward like a pendulum. When this swinging motion is inhibited, compensatory movement takes place somewhere else in the body. A chain reaction of unnecessary tensions travels throughout the structure to support the inappropriate motion. Instead of progressing smoothly forward, the weight of the body takes a lateral detour with each step.

The explorations in this chapter will help you restore the

independent motions of your pelvis and your femur (the thigh bone), so that these two parts of your hip joint can remember how to function in relationship rather than as a structural unit. In the scripts, you'll be directed to make some very small movements in very slow motion. The tiny movements are like secrets whispered to your nervous system, secrets about new ways of feeling and doing things. The nervous system is willing to entertain new possibilities when you whisper to it—it reacts by rote when you shout.

The slow-motion procedure induces relaxation of the surface layers of your musculature and teaches you to initiate movement from your core. The less active you are on the surface levels, the more you can feel what's happening at the core of your body. Once you've found ease at the core, you can move at any pace you like.

As you perform these patterns, you may notice little hesitations in your movement. This is a result of the neuromuscular responses along that movement path having become restricted by your habitual tension. Muscle fibers and their associated neurons are clumped together by your fascia, resulting in movement that jerks like the second hand on a battery-operated clock. By moving very slowly you give your system time to reorganize. As more fibers and neurons become operative, your movement becomes smooth, like the second hand on a spring-wound clock.

Releasing Your Inner Thigh

Script 10 explores the interplay of tension between the deep rotator muscles of the buttocks and the muscles and tendons of the inner thigh and groin. Tension in these muscles causes outwardly rotated feet and legs and restricts the free forward swing of the thighs.

You'll begin by lying on the floor barefoot with your knees bent, heels near your buttocks. Place a firm, thick cushion alongside one hip. Have your feet and knees about three inches apart from each other. Relax your leg muscles and let gravity support your bones. If your feet tend to slide away from your body when you start the exploration, you can lie with your toes against a wall.

The first motion of this script is to slowly lower one thigh onto the cushion at your side. Since you have at least eight cycles of breathing to complete the lowering process, you'll have plenty of time to release any increments of tension in your inner thigh muscles.

If releasing this tension makes you feel too vulnerable or anxious, continue breathing, and try to observe those feelings as if from a distance. The tension in your legs and hips may have been a way of protecting you from unwanted feelings in the past. With the calm flow of your breath, assure yourself that it is safe, in this time and place, for these muscles to relax.

The second part of script 10 helps you recognize the difference between raising your thigh with your buttocks tensed and hip joint compressed and raising it with your hip joint operating freely. While the first way may seem more familiar and easier, it actually requires more effort. If you relax your buttocks, gravity counterweights your knee and assists the inner thigh muscles in raising your leg.

Gravity is a great partner. You can recognize that gravity is supporting your structure when moving your body requires minimal muscular effort.

◆

SCRIPT 10

THIGH RELEASE AND LIFT

Lie with your knees bent toward the ceiling, feet slightly apart and close to your buttocks. Your knees should feel supported by your feet— don't let your knees lean on each other. Place a thick cushion beside your right thigh.

Tune in to the internal motion of your breathing, . . . the way your breath seems to flow through your body, . . . like a stream through mountain canyons. Be aware of the place where your lower spine joins your pelvis. Sense the movement of your breathing there. . . . It's like a place where the streambed widens.

Cup your palms around the curves of your buttocks. Picture the ball-and-socket joints inside; . . . feel them responding to the movement of your breathing.

In a moment, you're going to start letting your right thigh drift out to the right, and slowly lower it until it rests on the cushion beside you. As you do this, you'll notice the weight of your lower leg shifting to the outside edge of your foot.

Begin now, knowing you have at least eight full breathing cycles to reach your destination. Feel your buttock softening in your hand as the weight of your thigh passes through your hip joint. Your neck, jaw, and chest feel relaxed and comfortable as you focus your attention on the slow, slow release of your inner thigh.

You let the muscles along your inner thigh be passive, . . . let them rest against the large bone of your thigh. Your leg gets to take a vacation now. . . . At last, you entrust the weight of your leg to the cushion and to gravity.

Before making the long journey back to your starting position, you're going to explore an effortful, tense way of raising your thigh from the cushion. Start by contracting the muscles of your right buttock. With your palm cupped around your buttock, you can feel this clearly. As your buttock contracts, your inner thigh muscles tighten also, and you notice that your thigh begins to rise off the cushion. Go ahead and raise your knee upright, using these two sets of muscles.

And then, relaxing your thigh, slowly lower your leg onto the cushion once again. Take all the time you need, . . . smoothing out the little hesitations in the movement as your inner thigh releases.

This time, slowly raise your knee without tightening your buttock muscles. As your leg rises from the cushion, its weight settles back into your hip socket and onto the lateral edge of your foot. The motion is smooth and effortless, . . . as your knee slowly returns to the starting position, with its weight once again supported by the center of your foot.

Repeat this exploration for the left hip.

Differentiating
Thigh and Pelvis

Script 11 refines your awareness of the relationship between your thigh and pelvis. Your knees will be bent as before. Raising one knee, you'll draw tiny circles in the air with an imaginary marker on your kneecap. This attunes your neurology to subtle shifts of weight and changes of direction at your hip joint. The circles are minute, no larger than an inch in diameter, and the movement is so slow that an observer would assume your knee was still.

The motion of the knee results from subtle changes of direction at the hip joint, so focus your attention there. Imagine that your eyes and ears—all your senses—could be located inside the joint. This deep awareness will help free the joint's action. The more completely you can let go of unnecessary muscle contraction around the joint, the smoother your movements will be. If you feel discomfort in the crease of your groin—an indication that you are overworking your thigh muscles—try placing a hand lightly on the outside of your thigh in order to support the knee. Then, relax the groin muscles and let your thigh float in the hip socket. By sensitizing yourself to the subtlety available at your hip joints, you increase your capacity for responsive support in your pelvis.

SCRIPT 11

KNEE CIRCLES

Lie with your knees bent, heels close to your buttocks. Letting your right foot lift from the mat, raise your bent leg toward the ceiling until it finds a comfortable balance above your hip bone. Support your lower back by letting your left foot sink into the floor. Float your right knee above your pelvis like a compass needle seeking north. Soften the muscles of your inner thigh and buttocks, . . . soften the tendons across your groin, . . . relax your calf and foot.

In a moment, you're going to slowly draw a tiny circle in the air with your knee as if there were a magic marker on your kneecap. You'll direct this movement from inside your hip joint, turning the ball at the top of your thigh bone to move your knee. Make the circle about an inch in diameter, and let it take about six breathing cycles to complete.

Now, breathing easily, begin drawing your first circle. The more deeply you relax your groin and buttocks, the smoother the motion becomes. You can let go of any strain in your shoulders, jaw, or forehead. . . . Take another six breaths to circle your knee in the other direction. . . . Notice that at the top of the circle the weight of your leg can settle back into your pelvic basin. Let your lower back give in to this shift of weight.

When you've completed circling, release the tendons at your groin and let your foot drop back to its starting position.

Repeat this exploration with your left hip.

◆

Releasing the Hip Joint

Script 12 focuses your attention on what it feels like to let gravity direct the action of your hip and thigh. First you'll raise your knee to a place of balance above your groin. If you do this in a relaxed manner, you'll feel as though your thigh is falling upward into your pelvis. The place of balance is a zone rather than a single, static point. When poised there, your knee will feel suspended above your hip.

The second part of the pattern is to let go of the minimal tension remaining in your hip and let your leg fall back to where it started. For the few moments your thigh is falling, your hip joint operates without effort. This is a precious sensation. Plant this sensation like a seed in your neuromuscular garden. Soon you'll cultivate it in your walking as a swinging motion of your thigh through your hip joint.

◆

SCRIPT 12

FORWARD THIGH DROPS

Lying with your knees bent, lift your right heel from the floor. Your knee begins moving toward the ceiling. By letting your toes come off the floor, your knee continues moving upward, gradually arcing above your right hip. As you do this, sink your left foot gently into the floor to support your lower back.

As your right knee approaches vertical, you can feel the top of your thigh bone sinking down into your hip socket. Find a place of balance for your thigh, . . . where the very slightest effort lets your knee balance in the air. Were you to let go of that slight effort, your foot would drop back onto the mat.

Imagine a magnet affixed to the sole of your foot. The magnet attracts your foot to the floor. Releasing the tendons at your groin, your leg drops back to starting position. Try this action several times: raise your knee to the balance zone above your hip, . . . using the other leg as support, . . . then relax the muscles across your groin, . . . and let your foot drop back to the floor. Focus your attention on the moment when your thigh is "in flight." Remember what that moment of freedom feels like in your hip. You're going to find that feeling again in walking.

Repeat this exploration with your left leg.

$\blacklozenge$

Mobilizing Your Pelvis

Up to this point you've been focusing on the motion of your thigh in relation to your hip joint. This joint also allows the pelvis to move on the thigh if the lower spine is free. Both actions are necessary for the dynamic balance of your pelvis in walking. Script 13 helps you find motion in your lower spine.

For this exploration, you lie on the floor with your knees bent, feet close to your buttocks. The first action is to press the palms of your feet into the floor while exhaling. The pressure is too slight to actually be termed "pressure"—your legs should feel as though they are sinking into the ground, rather than being pushed with muscular effort.

As your feet sink down, you'll notice an adjustment in your pelvis—its weight begins rolling upward across your sacrum toward the small of your back. Have you ever noticed those dimples beside your sacrum? You'll feel your weight travel upward into those dimples. By letting your feet sink a little deeper, your pelvis can rise slightly up off the floor. This makes a hammocklike curve out of your lower back. Your abdomen relaxes, settling into the hammock.

The second part of the movement is to incrementally lower your sacrum to the starting position. At first you may feel that your sacrum can only come down in one chunk. If you go very,

very slowly, focusing your attention on your sacrum, you'll soon be able to appreciate tiny sensations that indicate your nervous system is rediscovering the precious movement within your pelvis.

The pelvic roll motion introduces the experience of subtlety to the deep muscles of the pelvis. These muscles are usually engaged in rigid reinforcement of the lower back, with all the muscle fibers firing at the same time, all the time. The pelvic-roll movement interrupts this pattern of "all or nothing" muscle tension and reminds the muscles of subtlety and differentiation. When these deep muscles recover their ability to move, tension in the lower spine is released.

An exercise called the pelvic tilt, a movement similar to the pelvic roll, is often taught in back-rehabilitation classes. In the pelvic tilt, you are taught to press your lower back into the floor by contracting your abdomen and then to lift your pelvis by tightening your buttocks and thighs. The goal is to build strength around a structural position that is believed to be correct. The Rolfing Movement approach is quite different. Rather than working to achieve a particular position for the pelvis, Rolfing Movement develops a new quality of motion within the pelvis. Range of movement—how high you lift your hips—is not important. The awareness is of *rolling* rather than *lifting*—as if your body fluids are being slowly poured upward through your trunk. When performed in this manner, your pelvis will rise without undue effort on the part of your buttocks, thighs, or belly. This insures mobility in front of the sacrum, an area of the spine that is usually immobile. Your sacrum, of course, does not actually roll—it is a sturdy plate of fused vertebrae. But by working with it as though it is flexible, you can coax responses from muscle fibers that don't ordinarily participate in movement.

The script for the pelvic roll teaches you to feel your weight shifting through an open pelvis with a flexible spine. You'll then be directed to perform the same motion the "wrong" way, with tension in your buttocks and thighs. This will demonstrate that tension in your hips reduces mobility in your lower spine. Though the action might look identical to an observer, the experience in your body will feel quite different.

At the end of script 13, you're invited to explore walking. You'll notice new mobility in your hip sockets—they'll feel smoother, as if they'd been lubricated. Your lower back and sacrum will be responsive to the movement of your legs as well as to the impulses of your upper body. You'll be riding along on an internal saddle, supported by your pelvis when you're in between one step and the next. The slight fluctuations of your pelvis give you a new relationship to gravity at each instant, adding fluency to your whole body's movement.

◆

SCRIPT 13

PELVIC ROLLS

Lie on the floor with your legs bent and feet slightly apart, so your knees are supported by your feet, . . . and turn your awareness to the motion of your breathing through the core of your body.

Next time you exhale, lightly press the palms of your feet into the floor, noticing how your pelvis rolls back as it adjusts to the shift of your weight. Letting your feet sink into the floor, feel your weight roll upward, . . . into the dimples beside your sacrum. This is a very small movement—just enough for you to feel a connection between your feet and your sacrum.

And exhaling once again, begin to reverse the motion, going very, very slowly, . . . noticing the smallest possible increments of movement, . . . as your sacrum rolls back down to rest.

This time, place the palms of your hands around the curve of your buttocks so your buttocks muscles stay soft as you repeat the upward roll. . . . Your abdomen relaxes too, . . . and you find a path for the movement behind your belly. This time let your feet sink a little deeper, so your pelvis rises ever so slightly from the floor. Your lower back lengthens, . . . and your abdomen feels as though it is settling back into a hammock.

And now, still breathing into your pelvis, . . . you unroll your spine, . . . down through the dimples, . . . slowly unfolding your sacrum, . . . as if laying down the links of a beautiful chain, . . . one tiny link at a time.

For contrast now, perform the motion a third time, letting your your inner thighs and buttocks contract as you roll your sacrum back down. Notice how the added tension reduces the feeling of flexibility in your lower back.

Release the added tension, and perform the motion one last time, with attention on the movement of the ball-and-socket joint inside your hips. You can feel this happening deep inside your buttocks when you let them relax. And as you slowly roll down your sacrum, you can appreciate the increasingly subtle sensations of movement within your pelvis.

If it seems comfortable, you can now let your legs slide down along the floor so you're lying fully extended. Slide a cushion under your knees.

Notice the feeling in your pelvis and legs right now. Find your own words to describe it. If you could hold that feeling in the palm of your hand, what would it look like? If it could make a sound, what would you hear?

Imagine what it would be like to walk with the feeling you have in your body right now. See yourself walking in this way. How is it different from the way you usually walk?

Now, begin returning to an ordinary state of awareness, bringing the new sensations with you. Let your eyes open, . . . and notice the shapes and colors around you. Feel the texture of the floor against your skin. Hear the sounds outside the room.

And, breathing easily, . . . let your pelvis continue to feel relaxed and spacious, . . . as you roll over onto your side, . . . and gradually push yourself up to sitting. And coming onto your hands and knees, . . . and onto your feet, . . . begin straightening your knees. And remembering to breathe into your core, . . . center your pelvis over the palms of your feet, . . . and slowly unfold your spine to standing.

Let the weight of your torso settle down through your pelvis and through your insteps into the earth. Let your pelvis feel open and spacious as you begin to walk. . . . Let your thighs swing easily. . . . The motion in your hip joints feels smooth and lubricated as your weight shifts smoothly from one foot to the other.

Notice any sensations in your knees or ankles that result from the improved mobility in your hips.

◆

You now have some experience of your pelvis as a relay station where your upper body weight shifts smoothly from one leg to the other as you walk, dance, work, or play. There are as many neuromuscular paths through the pelvis as there are human solutions to the task of walking. With your increased kinesthetic awareness, you'll be able to notice this variety of solutions as you watch other people walking. The most balanced neuromuscular path is through the center—a simple, fluid forward motion with no swivel, lurch, or sway. The pelvis should float between spine and legs, able to respond freely to moment-by-moment demands for support, balance, and expressiveness.

Familiarize your nervous system with your new pattern in small doses throughout the day. Perhaps there's a hallway or sidewalk that you walk along in the course of your daily routine. Let your presence in that specific place become a reminder of the new openness and support you're discovering in your pelvis. Take a breath, and for the length of the sidewalk, enjoy the ease of your new way of walking.

Spend several practice sessions becoming comfortable with the sensations and movements of scripts 10 through 13 before going on to the balance of this chapter. The last three scripts will take you to a deeper level of awareness of your pelvis.

Your Pelvic Floor

Script 14 incorporates awareness of the pelvic floor into the pelvic roll pattern. The pelvic floor is the triangular area defined by your sitting bones and pubic bone. It was introduced in chapter 3 as the base of support for your pelvis in balanced sitting.

The muscles of the pelvic floor form a divider or diaphragm that supports and controls both sexual activity and elimination. Needless to say, this is one of the most sensitive areas of the human body, neurologically intricate and intimately associated with experiences of human relationship. Whether from rude handling while being diapered as an infant, from confused feelings of adolescence, or from the atrocity of sexual abuse, the pelvic floor is a location of protective tension. Such tension can distort the structural balance of the entire body. As well, we've all been conditioned by our Judeo-Christian culture's denial or degradation of basic bodily functions. We're all victims of cultural abuse of the body.

Be patient with yourself as you develop your body image relative to your pelvis. You may feel vulnerable and even resist the awakening

BALANCING YOUR
BODY

sensations in this area of your body. Remember that your resistance is there to protect you. As you evolve other ways of protecting yourself, your physical tensions will no longer be needed.

Script 14 helps you develop a spacious pelvic floor and a broad base of support for your pelvis. It also helps adjust the angle or tilt of your pelvis.

Script 14 leads right into script 15, which reviews pelvic motion in the sitting position. It draws your attention to the sensation of motion in your hip joints and heightens your awareness of your internal saddle. For this exploration you'll need a chair with a firm seat. Adjust the chair's height so your hip joints are slightly higher than your knees.

◆

SCRIPT 14

PELVIC FLOOR EXPLORATION

Lying on the floor with your legs bent so your knees are supported by your feet, sense your breath moving throughout your body. Feel the pulse of your breath in your pelvic floor. As you soften the muscles around your sitting bones, . . . relaxing your genital area, . . . you can feel your pelvic floor expanding.

And now, as you exhale, . . . imagine your sitting bones being gently drawn toward your heels, . . . and lightly press the soles of your feet into the floor, . . . your pelvic floor begins turning toward the ceiling . . . Your pelvic floor remains soft and spacious as it rotates upward, . . . as your weight rolls back behind your soft belly and across your sacral dimples. Your calf and thigh muscles are relaxed, as your feet sink into the floor.

Now, breathing comfortably, . . . you reverse the pelvic roll motion, inwardly observing the movement of your pelvic floor as you return to your starting position.

For contrast, repeat the pelvic roll pattern, . . . but this time slightly contract the muscles of your pelvic floor. Notice how this makes your inner thighs and buttocks grip as well. This added tension reduces the mobility of your lower spine, compresses your hip joints, and diminishes the sensation of support from your feet.

Repeat the motion without added tension, breathing comfortably and taking all the time you need.

As you feel tensions in your pelvis receding, appreciate them for the protection they've provided you until now. As you let those shielding tensions go, know that they will be available if you ever need that protection again. Having choice is a wonderful opportunity. Appreciate the freedom that releasing these tensions brings you.

Slowly roll over onto your hands and knees. . . . Tuck your feet under and unfold yourself to a standing position, letting your pelvic floor remain spacious. Let yourself settle into the middle layer of your body with your weight centered over the palms of your feet. Be aware of your weight passing through your pelvic floor as you yield to the earth's support.

◆

SCRIPT 15

SEATED PELVIS EXPLORATION

Sit on a firm chair at the ideal height for your body, knees in front of you and heels directly below your knees. Be aware of how your feet and pelvis form a tripod that supports your body. Relax your pelvic floor, letting your pubic bone sink, and letting your weight settle into the internal saddle of your pelvis. Notice that the base of your spine is free to move.

Slowly rock your trunk forward across your sitting bones. Lean to an approximate sixty-degree angle, letting your head and torso follow the movement of your pelvis. Softening the muscle in the crease of your groin, . . . sense your weight traveling down through the core of your thighs and into your feet. Then use your feet to gently roll your weight back into the saddle, . . . keeping your groin and pelvic floor relaxed, . . . letting your torso unfold until you are sitting upright again.

And repeat the motion, gently rocking forward through your pelvic floor, letting your hips widen as your weight moves down into your feet. . . . And return, dropping through the palms of your feet and rolling into your pelvic saddle. And breathing comfortably, . . . rock forward again, . . . and back, . . . repeating the pattern several more times, becoming aware of the easy rotation in your hip joints, . . . as your pelvic basin rocks forward, . . . and back. Memorize the sensation in your hip joints, so you can find it again when you are walking.

◆

Gravity Game Reminder

Script 16 is an integrative movement pattern that helps your nervous system organize new information about your pelvis as a combination sling and saddle, about the way your core is supported by the centers of your feet, and about the balance between the impulses of push and reach. It's a simple knee bend performed very, very slowly to allow your neuromuscular apparatus time to coordinate all the new information.

Try a knee bend right now to evaluate how you would ordinarily do it. Stand comfortably, feet slightly apart and approximately in line with your nipples. Your sitting bones will be in line with your heels. In slow motion, simply bend your knees, letting the floor of your pelvis descend about two inches. Then slowly straighten your knees and come back to standing. Notice where you support your weight as you rise. Are your heels supporting your weight? Is there more tension in the back half of your body? Do you feel the impulse to rise as a reaching upward with your chest or as a pushing up from below with your legs? How are your pelvis and hips involved in this motion? What happens to the dimension of your pelvic floor?

When the movement is performed correctly, the pelvis will feel open and supportive, the core of the body will be centered over the arches of the feet, and, in coming up from the bent-knee position, the trunk will be raised by the pushing action of the legs.

If, during the walking evaluations in chapter 3, you noticed that you reach forward with your arms and chest in walking, you may have difficulty sensing the rising motion of the knee-bend pattern as a push into the ground. One way to find the push is to revise the way you think about it. Think of your relationship to gravity as a reach downward into the center of the earth—so, as your knees bend, you reach down through the centers of your feet. Continue the downward reach as you straighten your knees and rise. Those who tend to lead from the lower body already show a downward orientation. These people should find familiarity with the sense of the legs pushing into the earth.

The standing knee-bend pattern may be used as a Gravity Game reminder throughout the day. The sitting motion should be performed as a movement meditation rather than as an exercise. Practice in slow sets of three; three times in a row is a good dosage for your nervous system at any one time.

As it refines coordination and balance, the knee-bend pattern challenges the strength of muscles along the core of your body. It's typical to feel a characteristic shakiness when first exploring this pattern. This indicates that muscle fibers along a new pathway are being activated. The shakiness is like that of a newborn fawn trying to find its legs.

After three knee bends, you're invited to walk once more, to notice how the increased openness of your pelvic floor supports your movement. Just as you found three points of support in sitting—your two feet and your pelvic basin—you now have the same three points of support in standing and walking. And you'll be riding smoother in your "saddle."

You may well find that incorporation of the pelvic floor into your body image causes changes in distant parts of your body. How does your neck feel now that your pelvis is more open? your throat? your jaw? your solar plexus?

Recovery of support, balance, and responsiveness in your body depends upon having choice about your tensions. Usually our tensions are responses to a present stimulus that our nervous system confuses with a past trauma. The tensions are like shields that gave us beneficial and necessary protection back then but may be obsolete now. To replace them with balance and responsiveness may require some patience and courage.

The secondary tensions you find may represent unconscious concern for your safety as you let go of an ancient pattern of protection. Appreciate that response for its good intention. Take stock of your safety in the present moment. Let a feeling of safety be your guide for how much tension to release at any one time.

Should you experience anxiety in working with the pelvic-floor release patterns, or any of the explorations in this book, consult chapter 9 on personal processing. Should you continue to feel unsafe, please seek a professional body/mind therapist to help you sort through the emotions that arise. References are listed in the appendix.

SCRIPT 16

INTEGRATIVE KNEE BENDS

Stand with your feet comfortably apart, middle toes in line with your nipples, heels in line with your sitting bones. Let your weight settle into the palms of your feet, just in front of your heels. Invite your breath into all dimensions of your body: . . . front, . . . sides, . . . and back, . . . and let it flow through your core, . . . through your pelvic floor, . . . and down through your legs. And notice how your breath gently presses into the soles of your feet each time you inhale. And your feet can soften, . . . and widen, . . . and lengthen. Let your arms feel relaxed, . . . and your eyes gaze softly ahead, . . . so your head feels supported by your chest.

And, next time you exhale, let your knees soften as if you were beginning to squat. Moving in slow motion, let your knees bend, lowering your pelvic floor about two inches. As you sit down into your internal saddle, . . . your pelvic floor is spacious, your pubic bone released toward the floor, and your sitting bones heavy and wide apart. . . . Your weight settles down into the palms of your feet. You can feel your heart area supported by your pelvis, . . . and your pelvis supported by your feet.

And continuing to breathe, you rise by reaching down into the earth, . . . as your knees straighten very slowly, . . . letting the upper part of your body ride upward, supported by your pelvis. And should you notice yourself wavering back onto your heels, gently guide your weight through the palms of your feet instead.

Repeat this pattern two more times, timing it to your breathing cycle, one exhalation and inhalation to go down, and another cycle to come up. Bending your knees slightly, start to squat, releasing your pubic bone as your sitting bones widen. . . . And with awareness in the palms of your feet, . . . straighten your knees, rising through your middle layer.

Now you're ready to bring this new awareness of your body with you as you walk. Continue to let your pelvic floor be spacious, . . . feeling the width across your hips, . . . and stepping into soft, open feet, . . . your hip joints feel smooth, . . . as you ride along on your internal saddle. Your upper body, . . . and lower body move forward together, in harmony.

And you notice how comfortably your body supports your intention to move forward.

Find your own words to describe the sensation of walking right now. How does it feel in your pelvis and hips? How much of this feeling would be comfortable for you to take with you into your daily life?

Now stop walking, and imagine a dimmer switch inside your body. This switch gives you a way to adjust your internal feeling for just the right amount of new sensation in your pelvis. You can adjust the switch for more or less openness, depending on where you are and who you are with.

The Gravity Gang

Pelvises, as you know, come in an array of sizes, shapes, and spatial orientations. It's important to be aware of the spatial orientation of your pelvis as you work with the exercises in this chapter. If you are swaybacked, with your pelvis tipped forward, you'll have a different set of pelvic tensions than someone whose pelvis is tucked under. Pauline and Bill have some realizations, as they work with the pelvic scripts, that will help you in your own explorations.

Pauline, our singer friend, fits the swayback category. Her spine arches forward at the small of her back, and when she walks, she swivels her hips around that arched place. At first Pauline resists the hip-release patterns. "This is making my hips feel wider," she moans. For years she's been struggling with a tendency to gain weight in her thighs and buttocks, and no amount of exercise has slimmed them down.

Pauline persists with the hip patterns because her new awareness of support and dimension has already made such a difference in her singing. Maybe pelvic awareness will bring another surprise. But she grows even more frustrated as she attempts the pelvic rolls. "No way! My lower back feels like a brick wall," she mutters as she attempts to roll her weight slowly down through her pelvis from dimples to tailbone. "The sacrum is bone, isn' it? It can't unfold like links on a chain!"

Margie reminds Pauline to let the motion of her breathing flow through her body. While Pauline calms down, Margie puts on some soft music. "Imagine you're a mermaid," Margie suggests, appealing to Pauline's theatrical nature. "Your lower spine is the sensuous, glistening, silver tail of a mermaid."

Smiling, Pauline begins to relax. She realizes she's been unconsciously tensing her belly and, with a sigh, it releases. That old habit of trying to feel thin is so persistent. Now she can sense the fascial breathing motion in her sacrum. Picturing the movement of her silvery "tail," she's gradually able to roll slowly and smoothly down her sacrum. The first few times it makes her spine tingle pleasantly. Then comes a brief wave of anxiety.

"What's happening?" Margie asks, noticing the troubled expression on her friend's face.

"The strangest thing," Pauline replies, opening her eyes and sitting up. "Something I'd completely forgotten. When I was little, two or so, we used to visit my grandparents every weekend. It was a long drive, and my mom used to praise me for having a clean diaper all the way to Grandpa's. I remembered that just now—as if I could hear my mom saying it."

"Sounds like that might have something to do with the tension in your pelvis."

"I think so. The 'need to please Mom' buried down there under 'thinking thin.' Margie, this work is amazing!"

"It's like peeling off layers," Margie nods.

Pauline continues slowly rolling through her sacrum, experimenting with the sensations of release. Inwardly, she has a talk with her mother and with the little girl who tried so hard to be good.

"I don't have to do that anymore," she murmurs.

Margie watches a faint flush rise to Pauline's cheeks as her eyelids flicker open. Pauline smiles at her, brushing away a tear. "I'm okay," she says, answering Margie's questioning look.

When Pauline stands up to practice the knee-bend pattern, she has to concentrate hard to keep her abdomen and buttocks relaxed. Long ago, in a ballet class, she'd been taught to tuck her tail under by clenching her buttocks. Now she uses the mermaid image to help her lower spine lengthen as her knees bend. The more she relaxes her buttocks, the smoother the movement becomes.

For Pauline, the newfound mobility in her pelvis and hips is a great revelation. Walking is a brand new experience of swinging her thighs from her hip sockets rather than swiveling her hips around her lower spine.

"It's a little strange having my legs this far apart," she comments to Margie. "It almost feels unladylike."

"But your pelvis feels freer, doesn't it?" Margie asks.

"It certainly does. I was walking on a tightrope before. This feels so fluid," Pauline raves. Not one for doing anything halfway, Pauline practices her new walk so much that her hips feel sore. "I must be using an entirely different set of muscles," she thinks. A light bulb goes on in her head as she realizes that maybe her hips were always heavy because she wasn't really using them. Now that she is, maybe they'll slim down after all.

"'Oh, that this too too solid flesh would melt'," moans Bill as he looks in the mirror. No one could accuse him of insincerity—he's been breathing faithfully every night, visualizing a core of golden light, and he's made himself the object of many jokes by changing his workstation to better suit his structure. He does feel better sitting at his desk, but over there in the mirror he's as scrawny looking and slumped as ever. "Okay, gravity, ol' buddy," he says, shaking his fist at the mirror. "The pelvis better be that missing link."

Bill has a tucked-under pelvis with outwardly rotated legs and a tendency to kick his heels forward as he walks. His lower back, which should have a slight forward curve, is practically flat. For Bill, the most important part of the pelvic-mobility exercises is to learn to release the deep muscles of his pelvic floor. In exploring the pelvic roll, his first instinct is to contract those muscles. But my tail is too far under already, he thinks, so that can't be right. He remembers that responsive balance requires minimal muscular effort. "Okay, then I'll pretend it's just my bones moving. No muscles at all."

He pictures his pelvis floating on water like the hull of a ship. This makes the movement feel entirely different. His sitting bones are no longer squeezed together. His pelvic floor is spacious. He's aware of a remnant of tension around the very tip of his tailbone. As he lets that go, his pelvis feels even more free.

Bill's next challenge is to transfer the free feeling to standing and walking. He's so used to supporting himself with the tension in his buttocks that relaxing them makes him feel swaybacked. He looks in the mirror at his profile. There's a slight curve in his spine now but not a sway. He looks again—his chest appears broader. Best of all, he's acquired buns. He'd always wondered how those other guys filled out their jeans. He arches his back even more. Ouch! That's too much. "Put the changes on a dimmer switch," he tells himself, "and dial in for comfort."

Watching himself in the mirror, Bill makes the new look alternately vanish and reappear. Just by gripping his sitting bones together, he can recreate the slumped and tucked-under profile. When he releases his sitting bones, not only does his chest rise, but his body weight automatically rocks forward toward the centers of his feet. Though unfamiliar, this new stance is more stable. And it makes him look like he's been working out at the gym.

When Bill tries the knee-bend exercise, he immediately feels his pelvic floor contract. It takes him several tries before he can bend his knees without gripping his buttocks. It helps if he lets his pubic bone drop as his sitting bones widen. Once he's found the squatting sensation, his new walking pattern develops quickly. The new orientation of his pelvis makes his knees swing straight ahead rather than to the side as they did before.

In retrospect, it seems he'd been walking like a duck. He likes the directness and confidence of his new gait. There are surprising sensations in his feet as well. He seems to be rolling over his feet now, so the balls of his feet are active. He has real feet now, instead of flippers. The new gait makes Bill feel ... he searches for the right description. *Powerful.* What do you know!

It doesn't take long for Pauline to begin telling Fred about the Gravity Game. She's so enthusiastic that he asks to see the book she's reading. He's up for trying anything that might get rid of the nagging pain in his back.

Fred has less success with the pelvic-release patterns than our other friends. It isn't that he can't sense the ease in his hip joints and mobility in his lower back. He can, and it all feels great—as long as he's lying down. He can even feel his chest responding to the pelvic-roll motion, like a wave rippling upward through the core of his torso. But as soon as he stands up, his back is tight again. He walks like he always has—heavy on his heels, chest high, arms swinging. He likes his walk. It's jaunty and energetic, the walk of an up-and-coming man.

Just for the fun of it, Fred exaggerates his gait, arching his back, swinging his shoulders, and bouncing from his heels to his toes. He glances at his reflection in the plate glass window: Hitler would have approved. "Guess I *could* have more than one way of walking," he mutters. "I certainly have more than one mood."

He stops and stretches, easing the stiffness in his spine and reflecting on his various moods. There's his "tough sales challenge" mood, his karate workout mood—he feels their rhythms in his body—those two are not dissimilar. Then there's his seductive mood. He grins, remembering how shy he used to be around women—not anymore. A karate buddy had dared him to enter that go-go contest. . . . He breaks into an undulating turn, then glides across the floor to some internal music. That had been quite a year.

Fred resumes walking in his normal manner now, trying to let different parts of himself be expressed in his gait. He slows down and shortens his stride, letting his hips spread out a bit. That makes a difference. He feels his weight settle into his core. "I got it," he mutters to himself. "This feels easier and, . . ." he frowns, searching for the right word, "more integrated. And I feel . . . how? quieter?"

Fred isn't sure he likes the new feeling. His body is more relaxed, especially in the hips, but it seems soft somehow, and it doesn't match his image of how a man should walk. He goes out to the kitchen for a drink and dials Pauline's number. Just because she's so enthusiastic about gravity doesn't mean these exercises are for him. He listens to the phone ring.

There *is* that crankiness in his lower back though. It always gets worse after a long drive. He's adjusted his car seat to a more upright position and filled in the bucket seat with a firm cushion for better support. These changes make sense to him, but they aren't solving his problem. Well, he'll keep practicing the pelvic roll—it makes his back feel better. And who knows, maybe he'll discover something else about his body as he keeps reading.

"Pauline? Hi. It's Fred. Listen, I have an offer you won't refuse—gravity watching. I got tickets for the Lakers. Are you free tonight? Great. Pick you up at seven."

CHAPTER 5

GOING WITH
THE FLOW

Have you ever observed the grace of animals in the wild? Maybe you watched a wild mustang galloping across a mesa in the high desert of New Mexico. Or you might recall seeing a documentary film about Africa that showed antelope streaming across the savanna and giraffe grazing in the bush. Visualize the movement— it's smooth, fluid, and direct, with no superfluous activity. Can you imagine human beings going about their business with as much harmony, efficiency, and grace?

The foundation for fluid movement of the body is structural balance and support. You've begun to evoke this in yourself by exploring the material in the previous chapters—the balance between front, side, and back dimensions; the feeling of being supported from below by feet and pelvis and from within by an internal core; the responsiveness of breath moving through your body; and the congruency of intention and action. These awarenesses give your body a lightness that you're beginning to recognize and, hopefully, to crave. The present chapter elaborates on these concepts and helps you develop the coordination that makes fluidity possible.

The coordination we're seeking is a different sort of coordination than that learned by dancers or athletes, whose grace is often specific to their art. While they may move elegantly on the stage or playing field, they can be as ungainly as the next person in their day-to-day movements. The coordination we're looking for makes gracefulness available to everyone, all the time.

Imagine yourself riding a thoroughbred horse. Feel how light, smooth, and coordinated the motion is. Then picture yourself on a broken old nag: a heavy and jarring ride, isn't it? Poor Nelly's spine seems unconnected to her shoulders and haunches. As she lurches from one leg to another, so do you. By contrast, the thoroughbred's gait has a shock-absorbing quality that supports you at every moment.

Take some time to watch an animal. If there are no horses in your paddock, the neighbor's cat will do. Notice that the slightest inclination of the neck or flick of the paw sends a subtle play of movement reverberating through the whole body. A slight shift of weight ripples outward like a pebble cast into a pond. You may have felt a hint of such responsiveness in your own body as you worked with some of the previous explorations. What you see as you watch a healthy animal move, or feel when you ride a thoroughbred, is harmonious joint movement. You sense all the joints moving in concert—nothing withheld and nothing extraneous added.

Hinges

To begin evoking the quality of harmonious joint relationship in your body, imagine that your joints are hinges. Sitting just as you are, explore the joints of your feet and legs with that idea in mind. Notice how your toes can move up and down. When all five toes flex together, the toe joints form a horizontal hinge across the ball of the foot.

Move your foot up and down from the hinge at your ankle. The ankle can rotate and tilt as well as flex horizontally, but the hinge action is its basic movement in walking.

Stand up on one leg, and swing your lower leg at the knee hinge and your thigh from your hip hinge. Then walk around and feel the four pairs of hinges operating. Notice whether one hinge seems more active than the others. If you motivate your walking from your pelvis and lean your torso back, you'll feel movement at your knees but have little sensation of the hinge action in your ankles and toes. If your gait is impelled by your upper body, you may be aware of a strong push from your toes but have little awareness of motion in your hip joints.

Initiating Movement
from the Core

Your musculature is arranged in layers around your skeleton, with the muscles closest to the bones being responsible for your most intimate relationship with gravity—here your balance is fine-tuned. In most of us, the core muscles are held taut as if balance were a static state rather than a continuing process of give-and-take.

When the core is immobile, movement is initiated in the outer layers of the body. Large muscles are used for small tasks. Most of us work much too hard at the simple activities of walking, sitting, bending, and rising. We use almost as much effort to flip a switch as to jack up a car. We contract our thighs to move our toes and tighten our buttocks to move our knees. No wonder life seems so stressful.

This chapter guides you in learning to initiate movement from the core of your joints by relaxing the overworked muscles of the exterior. Your hinges can move with minimal effort. You'll discover energy-saving locomotion and learn to engage your larger muscles only when they're needed. The interplay between a resilient core and a responsive exterior makes fluidity possible.

Your movements may seem jerky in your initial explorations. Move at the pace of a growing plant. You're freeing the movement potential at the core of your body—give your system all the time it needs to integrate the new patterns into your neuromuscular circuitry. Gradually your movements will become smooth.

Awakening Your Toes

Script 17 investigates the hinge at the ball of the foot. For this exploration, you'll sit on the floor with your back supported against a wall or a piece of furniture. Sit with your knees bent and your feet flat on the floor. Seat yourself upright over your pelvic floor. If your pelvis rolls back in this position, elevate it by sitting on a folded towel or thin telephone book. A lift of an inch or even less will tilt your pelvis to a better angle to support your upper body.

The pattern is simply to move your toes, all five together, slowly up and down. At first you'll find your leg muscles straining to raise your toes. As you learn to relax the exterior muscles and let gravity support your leg, effort gets pared to a minimum and the toes can move effortlessly from the core.

You may find that your baby toes tend to lag behind the others. By activating your baby toes, you'll develop strength along the lateral edge of your foot and broaden your base of support.

Practice the pattern with one foot and then the other, noticing differences in the way they respond. If one foot learns the new way of moving more readily, let it be the "teacher" for the other one to match its quality.

◆

SCRIPT 17

TOE-HINGE EXPLORATION

Sit on the floor with your knees bent, your back against a wall or a sturdy piece of furniture. Situate your pelvic basin right under your trunk. A slight lift under your buttocks can make you more comfortable in this position.

Starting with your right foot, raise your toes off the floor. Place your right hand along your shin so you can feel your leg muscles contracting as your toes are raised. Move your toes up and down several times. In addition to feeling your leg muscles contract, you may even sense some effort in your thigh. In a few minutes you'll discover a way of raising your toes without this unnecessary effort.

Relax your toes now, and turn your attention to your breathing for a few moments. Remind yourself of the way your fascia responds to your breathing. Let the muscles of your legs soften, . . . let them rest on the bones. Imagine your breath flowing through the core of your right leg and down into your foot. Notice the weight of your leg resting on your foot.

Now you're going to raise your toes with the least possible amount of effort. With your hand still resting on your shin, let your right foot settle even more deeply into the floor, . . . so deeply that your foot seems to be getting longer, . . . and now, as you exhale, your toes begin rising from the floor, . . . uncurling as they rise, . . . their delicate undersides lengthening. Then slowly relax your toes, . . . letting them stay long as they return to the floor.

Repeat this motion with attention on your baby toes. Let your fourth and fifth toes lead the way up. Notice the activity along the outside edge of your foot when your baby toes participate. Continue breathing easily. Soften the muscles of your calf, thigh, neck, jaw, and eyes. Your toes can move slowly up and down on their hinges while the rest of your body rests.

Carefully repeat this process for your left foot.

◆

Articulating Your Feet

Script 18 helps you initiate foot action from the core, without unnecessary contraction of shin or thigh muscles, and coordinate the hinges at toe and ankle. It's true that if you tighten the outer muscles of your shin and thigh, you can achieve greater range of motion at the ankle joint than you can in the relaxed fashion suggested here. However, with these exercises we're developing integrated joint action rather than extreme range of motion in any single joint. By inhibiting the habitual strong contraction, you make way for the emergence of a new neuromuscular pattern.

◆

SCRIPT 18

TOE AND ANKLE INTEGRATION

Sit with your back against a wall, your knees bent, feet flat on the floor, and calf and shin muscles relaxed. Lengthening the undersides of your toes, . . . and leading with your baby toes, gently raise the toes of your right foot. . . . Now slowly flex your right ankle, calf and shin still soft, pivoting your heel so that your toes and the sole of your foot rise off the floor. . . . Then, relaxing your ankle, . . . slowly return your foot to the floor, setting the toe hinge down first, . . . then gently lowering your toes. The palm of your foot feels very long and wide and open.

Slowly repeat this movement with quiet attention on the breath. As you exhale, your toes come up, . . . and your foot comes up, . . . the palm of your foot opening. . . . Then gently inhale, . . . and as you exhale again, your toe hinge returns to the floor, . . . the palm softening, . . . and then your toes return to the floor.

As you repeat the motion once again, notice that when you raise your foot onto the heel, your knee responds to the ankle motion by passively bending, . . . and your thigh bone passively rotates in your hip socket. Pause with toes in the up position, and notice the weight of your leg resting on your heel and your sitting bone. . . . Let all your leg muscles rest on the bridge of bone suspended between these two points. . . . Then slowly relax your ankle and return your foot, . . . and your toes, . . . to the floor.

Repeat these patterns with your left leg.

◆

Integrating Ankle, Knee, and Hip Hinges

Script 19 coordinates the hinges at ankle, knee, and hip. The movement is similar to the ankle flexion pattern in script 18, except that you begin with your working leg extended. Bending ankle and knee at the same time, you flex your foot and let your knee rise toward the ceiling. Your heel stays on the floor as if glued to its original spot. The upper and lower segments of your leg rise from the floor like the two sides of a drawbridge. When the ankle is fully flexed, the weight of the leg will be resting on two points: the heel and the sitting bone.

The tricky part of this coordination is to avoid contracting the upper thigh muscles to bend the knee. To avert this tendency, script 19 begins by reviewing the ankle-flexion pattern, with your foot placed progressively farther away from your body each time.

Once you're familiar with the drawbridge pattern, you'll compare this relaxed hinging of your joints with a similar movement initiated by your thigh muscles. When you perform the action the second way, you'll feel your leg shortening as if it were being sucked up into your hip joint. You'll also sense the absence of participation by your ankle and toe hinges. Relaxing your thigh and groin again, you'll feel your leg lengthen and all four hinges come back into play. When the movement is performed correctly, the ankle starts the action, the knee bends passively, and the thigh stays relaxed.

◆

SCRIPT 19

THE DRAWBRIDGE

Begin by sitting against a wall with both knees bent. Slide your right foot about five inches farther away from your hips, and place your right hand lightly on your thigh. Repeat the ankle-flexion movement from script 18, letting your toes be relaxed this time. Notice the weight increasing in your right heel and sitting bone as your foot rises. Your knee bends passively; your thigh muscles stay soft because the movement is directed by your foot.

Slide your foot out another five inches and repeat the pattern. This time let your ankle and knees bend as you exhale. Your thigh muscles continue to feel soft under your hand.

Now extend your right leg all the way out in front of you. With your heel holding its place on the floor, let your ankle bend again, . . . and as your toes move toward your knees, your knee passively rises toward the ceiling. The weight of your lower leg rests into your heel, . . . and the weight of your upper leg rests into your sitting bone. Your leg bends in the middle like a drawbridge.

Breathing comfortably, lower your leg by relaxing your ankle and lowering your foot. Notice any remaining tensions in your body and release them.

For contrast with this relaxed way of coordinating your ankle, knee, and hip hinges, initiate the same action by contracting your thigh muscles. . . . Notice that the crease at your groin tightens and your leg feels shorter, as if pulled into your hip sockets. Very little weight rests on your heel. . . . Now relax your effort and return your leg to the extended position.

Breathing comfortably, let your thigh muscles soften once again, . . . until your leg feels heavy and completely supported by the floor. Gently adjust your leg so your kneecap faces upward to the ceiling. Now, as the weight of your leg drops into your heel and sitting bone, . . . the draw-bridge starts to come up again: . . . your ankle flexes, . . . and with soft thigh muscles, . . . and soft groin muscles, . . . your knee rises.

And when your ankle relaxes, your leg returns to the floor. Notice how much longer your leg feels now.

Repeat this pattern with your left leg. Notice differences in the way each leg responds. If one leg has more difficulty with this pattern, spend a little extra time exploring on that side.

◆

Combination Patterns

Script 20 is a combination of the patterns explored in scripts 12 and 19. First you'll practice the drawbridge pattern lying down. Then you'll drag your heel all the way up to your buttock, letting your foot come up from the floor until your knee is over your pelvis. You finish by releasing the groin and dropping the thigh. In combination these patterns increase the coordination of the joints of your leg.

◆

SCRIPT 20

DRAWBRIDGE, DRAG, AND DROP

Lie on your back with your left leg bent, foot flat on the floor. Your right leg is extended long from the hip joint. Follow your breathing for several cycles, . . . enjoying the pause at the end of each exhalation. You can feel your whole body respond internally as the air goes in and out. Pay special attention to the movement of your breath in your lower spine. . . . Let your breath soften and widen the area around your sacrum.

And as you let the weight of your right leg settle into your right heel and sitting bone, . . . your ankle begins to bend, . . . your instep rises toward your knee, . . . and your knee bends toward the ceiling. . . . Feel the weight of your thigh shift upward through your hip joint and back into your pelvis. Extend your leg again by softening the muscles at the back of the leg, . . . softening your ankle, . . . and letting the ball of your foot move downward. . . . Slowly repeat this pattern.

Bring the drawbridge up a third time, pausing at the top. Apply slight pressure against the floor with your left foot to support your lower back. Now, relaxing your raised calf and foot, draw your knee toward the ceiling, dragging your heel along the floor. As your thigh approaches vertical, your foot will rise from the floor. Let your knee continue to rise in an arc over your pelvis until it finds a place of balance. Feel your leg being supported in the hip socket by your pelvis. . . . Feel your pelvis being supported by gravity.

In a moment, you're going to relax your groin muscles and let your leg drop to the floor. Imagine there's a magnet on the sole of your foot. When you're ready, release your groin muscles and let the magnet pull your foot down. Your hip joint relaxes as your leg falls.

Pause now, with both legs bent, . . . reminding yourself to breathe, . . . and releasing any tension that may have crept into your neck, shoulders, abdomen, or jaw. Then slowly slide your left leg down to an extended position. And repeat the pattern—drawbridge bending, . . . leg dragging upward, . . . balance, . . . and drop.

Alternate your legs several times, noticing whether one side seems to catch on to the pattern more readily. Let that side teach the other one how to do it. Notice how the side that is not working supports the moving side. Each side needs support from the other.

◆

You'll complete your exploration of hinges with a review of the pelvic roll, roll up to standing, and standing knee bends. You'll find that your new awareness of fluid joint motion deepens your experience of these patterns from previous chapters. Script 21 directs your review of these patterns.

SCRIPT 21

PELVIC ROLL, ROLL TO STANDING, KNEE BENDS

Lying on the floor with both knees bent, relax your calves and let their weight be supported by your feet. Relax your thighs and let their weight be supported by your pelvis. Notice your breath moving through the middle layer of your body,... from your feet all the way through your legs,... pelvis,... torso,... and head.

And on your next exhalation, let your sitting bones migrate downward toward your heels,... as your buttocks soften,... and your insteps settle deeper into the floor. You can feel your pelvic floor turning toward the ceiling,... as your weight shifts back across the dimples beside your sacrum,... and into your lower back. Relaxing any tension around your sitting bones and buttocks,... you can feel the spaciousness of your pelvic floor. And when you gently press into your feet,... your weight travels up your spine into your rib cage,... a river flowing northward through your body.

As you exhale, you slowly reverse the direction,... letting your weight settle down through your lower back,... sacrum,... thighs, ... and feet.

If your eyes have been closed, let them open now,... and become aware of your surroundings. When you're ready, gently roll to one side and then onto your hands and knees. Position your knees in line with your nipples. Tuck your toes under, and push your weight back onto your feet,... letting your neck relax so your head dangles. As you exhale, rest into the centers of your feet and let your knees extend, your upper body still hanging forward. With your knees straight but not locked, turn your pelvic basin until it is level,... allowing your torso to rise. Continue breathing,... and with your weight still centered over your insteps,... slowly unfold the twenty-four hinges of your vertebral spine:... lower spine,... thorax,... upper spine,... neck,... and head.

Standing comfortably, breathe into all dimensions of your rib cage, ...front,... side,... and back. Relax your buttocks muscles, feeling the spaciousness of your pelvic floor. Now slowly bend your knees as if you were starting to squat. Your pelvic floor lowers about two inches. As you lower your weight through the palms of your feet, feel how the earth supports you. Notice how your ankle, knee, and hip hinges bend in unison. As you exhale, reach down through your feet and slowly rise, . . . feeling the hinges extending and pushing your torso upward.

Repeat the knee-bend pattern. . . . Your upper body rides down as if on an elevator, . . . and then is borne up from below as your knees straighten. The earth supports you all the way down, . . . and all the way up.

◆

Internal Suspenders

Responsive movement of the lower spine and pelvis and free swinging of the thighs in walking depend on the release of specific core musculature called the iliopsoas. This muscle group lies along the lower spine from the diaphragm down to the pelvis. It passes diagonally through the pelvis, crosses the groin, and connects to the top of the inner thigh. This very important core structure should function like internal suspenders connecting spine and legs. The iliopsoas performs two functions—it tilts your pelvis as in the pelvic roll (script 13, page 76) and it contributes to the pendulum motion of the legs in walking.

Most people sense their legs originating at the tops of the thighs. When the iliopsoas muscles operate freely, the legs feel as though they begin higher up and in the core of the body, just under the rib cage.

Script 22 helps you discover and release your suspender muscles. For this exploration, you need a small, sturdy stool or pile of telephone books three to four inches high. You'll stand with one foot on this platform and let your other leg swing from its suspender. Once you've felt the core suspension of each leg, you'll find that walking feels very different, as if your legs are swinging down *through* your pelvis. Memorize this sensation. Later on, just remembering it will be enough to evoke the change in your walking.

SCRIPT 22

ACTIVATING YOUR
SUSPENDER MUSCLES

Put your platform in a doorway and place your right foot on the edge of the platform. Lightly rest your hands on the doorjamb for security, and step onto the platform, letting your left foot clear the edge. Stand high on your right leg, keeping your hips level. Let your left leg relax into a gentle swing, . . . forward two or three inches and back. The pendulum swing takes almost no effort. Feel the ball-and-socket joint rotating freely deep inside your buttocks. Relax the upper part of your torso, and breathe.

Imagine a suspender attached just behind your respiratory diaphragm. Your hanging leg is suspended from here. The suspender dangles down through your pelvis. As your leg swings, you can feel the reverberation up through your hip joint, pelvis, and rib cage. Imagine the motion of your leg beginning just below your ribs.

Now turn around and stand with your left leg on the box. Be sure that your hip joints are horizontal and that you're not sinking into your left hip. Use your hands for support on the door frame. And let your right leg swing, . . . relaxing your buttocks, . . . breathing, . . . finding that suspender up under your rib cage, . . . feeling your swinging leg getting longer, . . . as it drops down through your hip joint.

Now step down from your platform and explore walking. Your legs now hang from your rib cage. Each leg swings easily down through your pelvis, . . . as your thighs take turns, . . . sending your weight through your knees, . . . into the soft centers of your feet.

Memorize this sensation, so you can find it again whenever you wish.

◆

Fluid Walking

How do you walk now that you've lubricated your hinges? Walk around the room for a while, contemplating the various sensations you've become aware of in the preceding chapters.

By this time you're recognizing the core of your body as your internal home, the place where your movement originates. The outer dimensions of your body image are configured around this core.

The interplay of your core and peripheral movements is supported from below by your pelvic floor and by the palms of your feet. With every footfall, your structure finds a soft foundation in your feet. You roll across the resilient palms of your feet from heels to balls. Your toe hinge helps propel you into the next step, and you glide forward across responsive ankles.

Your legs feel long, as though they're suspended from the middle of your spine. They hang down through your pelvis, your thighs swinging like pendulums. Your pelvis seems to float between your hip joints and your spine, a gently fluctuating saddle that supports you as you ride along.

Your locomotion is the result of congruent impulses of your gut, heart, and head. You no longer have to reach with your upper body or push with your pelvis. Instead, all of you moves forward together. You spend the same amount of time on the leg that strides forward as on the one that pushes from behind. The concerted action of your leg hinges makes your progress smooth. While your gait may not yet match this description in every detail, you have achieved enough change and choice in your movement that you know more comfort is just a matter of time.

Getting in Stride

Practice walking in a contemplative way for a few minutes every day, evoking in yourself the qualities you found by exploring your hinges. Experiment with the length of your stride. For many people, shortening the stride slightly can improve both support and fluidity. If you're small in stature or if you have a significant other who is tall, it's likely you're taking long steps to keep up with your companions. Those big steps may be undermining your best relationship to your own body. Try shortening your stride by half a toe's length. That's not much, but it can make a big difference in your support system.

Develop flexibility in your gait so that you can at least claim support and comfort for yourself when you're walking alone. If you must keep up with a tall person, try doing so by taking a greater number of shorter steps rather than by matching her rhythm. Initially this may make you feel like you're mincing along, but that's only because it's unfamiliar, or perhaps because of some belief you have about how a "real man" or "real woman" ought to move. Reevaluate your beliefs. Determine their effects on your body's comfort. If you persevere with the explorations in this book, you'll become accustomed to fluid motion. It can become addicting because it feels so good.

The width of your stride is another factor that influences both your support and your fluidity. Some people walk with their legs too close together, as if they were on a tightrope. Although a narrow base may be pleasing aesthetically, its maintenance requires excessive tension in the inner thighs and pelvic floor. In general, good use of human structure has the knees lined up under the nipples, not under the navel.

A wide base can be appropriate for certain types of activities such as practicing martial arts or lifting heavy loads. But when the legs are too far apart in walking, they can't provide adequate support for the center of the trunk. The result is excessive tension in the core of the body. People with this pattern tend to sway from one leg to the other, like frequenters of the OK Corral.

Should your base be either too wide or too narrow, review the hip-release and pelvic-floor patterns in chapter 4 and standing knee bends in chapter 3. If your base is narrow, put your attention toward releasing your inner thigh muscles and keeping your pelvic floor spacious. When practicing the knee-bend pattern, imagine that just as your pants have inseams and outer seams, so do your legs. As you bend and straighten your legs during the knee bend, relax the inseams of your legs so they're just as long as the side seams. This image is also helpful in practicing the drawbridge pattern and in walking as well.

If your base is wide, release your buttocks and cultivate the sensation of mobility in your hip sockets. Let the outer line of your legs relax and lengthen as you walk.

The best guides for determining appropriate stride length and width are the sensations of support and fluidity. Rather than relying on a visual image of correct movement, let the good feeling, the sense of ease, be your guide. If you stay attentive to sensation, you'll evolve good use of your structure from the core outward. On the other hand, if you imitate an idealized picture, you're likely to add an inauthentic pattern to your old habits.

Best Feet Forward

Few of us pay much attention to our feet until they begin to hurt. One of the most troublesome things is the development of a bunion or enlargement of the joint at the base of the big toe. While this may be worsened by ill-fitting shoes, the basic cause is poor structural use of the feet. If you've noticed such a bump developing, take a look at how you're using your feet. You'll find that you're walking with your feet turned out. Instead of moving in a straight line through your foot, your weight travels from the outside edge of your heel diagonally across the sole of your foot to the big-toe joint. During the pushing phase of your stride, you put so much pressure on the big-toe joint that the big toe is pushed inward toward the other toes.

If the bunion is far advanced, movement reeducation won't reverse it but can prevent it from getting worse. Practice the toe-hinge motions (script 17, page 92) with special attention on your fourth and fifth toes. This helps activate support from the lateral edge of your foot and de-emphasizes your reliance on the big-toe joint.

Often the turned-out position of the foot is the result of outward rotation of the thighs or is compensation for inward rotation. Aligning the hip and knee hinges will set your feet on the right track. Practice the hip release patterns in chapter 4 (script 10, page 70; script 11, page 72; script 12, page 73, script 13, page 76) and the patterns for integrating ankle, knee, and hip (scripts 18 and 19, pages 93 and 95).

In the standing knee-bend exercise and in walking, you may be tempted to force your feet into a parallel position. Even though your eventual goal is for your feet to track forward, forcing your legs into this position would be too immediate a change and would cause strain and discomfort in your knees. Instead, focus on pointing your kneecaps forward. As your hips become freer, your knees will communicate the change to your feet.

Many people have been told that they have flat feet. This usually means that the muscles of the sole of the foot are not properly developed. Walking as you have been learning in these explorations, with the body balanced over the centers of the feet and toe and ankle hinges fully articulating, will strengthen underdeveloped arches and may even eliminate the need for arch-support shoes.

If the Shoe Fits

The appropriateness of shoes in general can be judged by their ability to let your weight fall centered and your feet articulate fully. Thong sandals tend to make you scuff your feet in order to keep the sandals from falling off. When you shuffle, you automatically kick your knees forward and lean your upper body back. If you must wear thongs, at least avoid wearing them for long stretches of time.

So-called health sandals with a recessed heel also tend to shift your body weight backward. The design of the shoes is meant to relieve back strain by lengthening the lower spine. For people who tend to lean forward and who have forward-tipped pelvises, the negative heel may have the desired effect. For those whose pelvises tuck under, the result is that the head projects forward to compensate for the weight thrust back into the recessed heels. This causes unnecessary strain in the neck. If you already own a pair of these sandals, which are too expensive to discard, I recommend filling in the negative heel with foam padding.

Consistent wearing of high heels is undesirable for two reasons. First, the shoes throw your weight forward. When this occurs, something somewhere else in your body has to shift back. Your body compensates in one of two ways—by exaggerating a sway in the lower back or by tucking the tail under and collapsing the upper chest. If your structure already exhibits either of these patterns, wearing high heels will make it worse.

The second strike against heels is that they virtually immobilize your toe and ankle hinges. You might as well put your feet in casts. The result is that other joints must work harder to get you where you're going. Added movement in your knees may cause no problem, but swiveling your pelvis around your lower back, which is the other compensatory action, will cause structural problems down the line. Enjoy wearing heels for power dressing and parties if you like, but do choose more structure-friendly shoes for all the other activities of your life.

Old shoes with worn heels can also undermine your support. Check your shoes: if the heel is severely worn on the outside edge, the shoe will prevent you from moving through the center of your foot by keeping your ankle hinge tilted laterally. An imbalanced shoe constantly reinforces your old walking pattern.

One of the nicest things people can do for their feet is abandon shoes all together. Kick them off and walk barefoot in sand or soft grass. Feel the grass between your toes. Give your feet some sensual pleasure. They're hard workers—they deserve some pleasure and rest.

Rotary Motion

Needless to say, there are many situations where an activity demands that a joint function other than as a simple horizontal hinge. Fortunately, we're not constructed like the Tin Man, and we do have rotational possibilities in our hips, ankles, and feet, though less so in our knees. We'd be sadly out of luck on a ski slope, tennis court, or dance floor if we were incapable of rotary motion in our lower limbs. The alignment of horizontal hinges along a vertical core is just a metaphor for the basic balance of the human structure. It's a map to your home in gravity.

Every Chair Is a Rocker

There are as many ways to get from sitting to standing as there are chairs and bodies. Most chairs are ill-fitted to the bodies they're meant to support. And most people get themselves from down to up without much awareness of the process. The usual approach is to attempt to rise straight up by reaching forward with the chest and then hoisting the torso up with the back half of the trunk. The legs are engaged almost as an afterthought.

In script 23, the emphasis is on the front half of the body and on the legs. You learn to get up by rocking down first and letting gravity rebound you upward. For this exploration, you'll need a firm chair or bench, adjusted to an ideal height for your frame.

Your hip joints should be slightly higher than your knees.

The exploration has four stages. First, you'll get used to the shift of weight between your pelvis and feet by just rocking forward and back. The next stage has you pitching forward until your torso is hanging upside down over your feet. In the third stage, you unfold your spine from the upside-down position. Your head and chest ascend by being pushed upward from below.

Once these three actions are smooth and easy, you'll learn to let the momentum ride through the core of your body. As the rocking movement becomes more refined, you develop a more socially acceptable way of standing up.

Get ready for a little comedy because the learning steps lead you through some anthropoid stages. But evolution toward a more comfortable use of your structure will be worth making a monkey out of yourself.

◆

SCRIPT 23

MOVING FROM SITTING TO STANDING

Sit on a firm chair at a height that allows your hip joints to be slightly higher than your knees. Your feet are resting on the floor. Your thighs face forward, and your heels are just beneath your knees. Let your arms hang beside your torso, hands relaxed beside your thighs.

Slowly rock your body forward across your sitting bones, . . . letting your upper body and pelvis ride forward together, . . . relaxing your neck so your head nods down, . . . and relaxing your shoulders so your arms hang loose. Pause when your torso leans to about a sixty-degree angle. Feel your weight supported by the tripod of feet and pelvis.

Now press down on your feet to roll your pelvis back to level, . . . and let your spine unfold to upright.

Repeat the forward-rocking motion, going a little farther down this time and letting your weight shift into your legs and feet as your torso descends. Now push through your feet to roll your weight back into your pelvis and up your spine. Be aware of your relationship to gravity as you again rock forward, . . . and roll back.

Now move one foot back so the heel is just below the edge of the chair. This time as you rock forward, allow your momentum to take you onto your feet, ... and let your upper body hang relaxed, head down and arms dangling. The back half of your body is relaxed, ... resting on the front half. For a moment you hang suspended at a point of dynamic balance. Then let your pelvis drop back onto the chair, ... and unfold your torso, neck, and head until you are sitting upright again.

Once again, rock forward, ... hanging upside down like a chimpanzee, ... rock back to the chair, ... and roll up.

This time, just as you reach the point of upside-down balance, reach down into the earth with your feet. As your knees straighten, your pelvis is pushed upward and your spine unrolls to standing. Your weight is over your front foot, so you're ready to take a step forward.

To sit down again, reverse the action: drop your head forward and bend your knees so you drop straight down over your forward foot. When your torso is hanging upside down, let your weight shift back across your back foot and drop your pelvis onto the seat. Then unfold your spine to upright.

Understanding that this stylized way of standing up and sitting down is not yet a seamless movement, explore the motion several more times. Focus your attention on your relationship to gravity, on the moment when your momentum thrusts you upward.

To stand, rock your torso forward, ... falling upside down over your feet, ... pushing down into the earth, ... and your knees straighten, ... pelvis rises, ... torso unfolds.

To sit down, roll your head forward, ... bend your knees, ... and your weight descends over your forward foot. Once you're upside down, let your weight shift back across the back foot, ... drop your pelvis onto the seat, ... and unroll your spine.

Notice that your upper body goes along for the ride in both standing up and sitting down. Focus your attention on the coordination of your leg hinges and pelvis as you perform the action once more. The upper half of your body moves because it's attached to the lower half. Notice also that the back of your body is relaxed, resting on the front.

Now you're ready to evolve a more socially acceptable way of standing and sitting. You're going to reduce the exaggerated folding and unfolding of your spine, and instead of falling all the way forward onto the front half of your body, you'll let your momentum travel upward through your core.

This time as you rock forward onto your feet, let your upper body start to rise just before it begins to fall. Your torso unfolds and your *knees straighten, taking advantage of your forward momentum. Your head makes only a slight dip as you rock forward and then is righted by your upward momentum. Gravity fully supports your rise through the central core of your body.*

The Gravity Gang

"It's incredible," Margie pants, sitting herself down at the café counter. The morning rush has settled, so Pauline has time for a chat. Though brimming with her own news, Margie notices something unusual about Pauline. She looks calm. She's been serving breakfast since 6 A.M. and usually by 9 she's a wreck.

"Did Steve hire more help for the morning shift?" Margie asks, looking around.

"Nope. But I did get some help," smiles Pauline. "And you look like you swallowed a canary. What's got you purring so excitedly?"

"Well," Margie replies, "this morning I decided to pay attention to my hinges while I was out on my run, and I discovered how to use my toes. I thought I had my weight over my feet before, but I guess I was still moving on the outside edges. Once I got my feet in gear, it felt like I was running on a rebounder, or flying on a magic carpet!"

"Gravity gave me some extra energy this morning too," Pauline says, setting a glass of orange juice in front of her friend. "Margie, I'm so glad we decided to do this movement program together."

"Me too." Margie sips her juice thoughtfully. "I never realized how much I was swaying from side to side until suddenly I wasn't swaying anymore. Now I can just move forward without any extra commotion."

"You know, we get our cars aligned every so often, it makes sense that our bodies work better if they're aligned too."

"I know. Moving this way makes me feel so light."

"I've seen some light myself," laughs Pauline. "You know how paranoid I've been about my thighs? Well, I had a hard time with those hinge patterns because the book said to let your legs feel soft and heavy. I was about to throw that book through the window."

Margie nods sympathetically. She's glad they have some time to talk while their impressions are fresh.

At the moment, the café is nearly empty of customers, so Pauline sits down next to Margie. "But then," she continues, "I had a hunch that if I went *through* the heaviness, I might find something else. So I kept on. When I lay down to do the integration pattern, I started crying—for no reason it seemed, except letting go of my legs somehow felt sad. But I remembered what Bill told us about the time when he got panicky doing the breathing exploration, how he watched himself like a spectator. So I just watched myself feel sad. As I did that, I realized that my legs didn't feel heavy so much as dense. Like I was tensing them up without being aware of it. And then I remembered the braces I had to wear when I was in first grade."

"What was wrong?"

"I was kind of knock-kneed. I only wore the braces for about a year, but I hated it. I think I just sort of abandoned my legs then and never came back, . . . I just withdrew my feelings from my legs. Maybe the sadness was about having been gone so long."

"But you're back now," Margie says softly. "What happened next?"

"The next part was the pelvic roll, and when I did that I felt an amazing tingling sensation in my hip sockets, as if they were waking up. My pelvis felt like it was floating. It still does, and now I *know* I'm going to lose these saddlebags at my hips!"

"No wonder you look so chipper on a Thursday morning," comments Margie. "It's a paradox, isn't it? that motion in your pelvis should make you feel so supported? You'd think your hips would feel more secure if they were locked in place."

"All I know," Pauline says, "is that if I stay in contact with my core, I can move fast without hurrying. I've never felt so at home, so at peace in my body."

CHAPTER 6

WINGS TO FLY

How would it feel *not* to have tension in your shoulders? For many people, such a possibility is unimaginable. Our evolutionary ancestors swung from trees as their primary means of locomotion, an activity that would have released any superfluous tension from their shoulder girdles. In contrast, our sedentary lifestyles rarely call for using the full range of motion available to the shoulders. Since we don't use that range, our muscles and fascia obligingly shorten.

Shoulder tension can be protective, retracting your head and chest like a turtle to shield you from life's buffeting. It can be motivating, squaring your shoulders for that drive to the finish. Or it can be supportive, compensating for structural deficiency lower down in the body. The discomfort that accompanies shoulder tension is a message from your body that you need to get your support or protection in some other way. The goal of this chapter is to help you find ease and competence in your upper body so that discomfort in your shoulders will be a thing of the past.

A Map of the Shoulders

Your shoulder girdle is made up of four bony parts: two shoulder blades and two collarbones. Your shoulder blades are triangular plates that should lie flat along the back of your rib cage. They're attached to your spine from their inside edge by sheets of muscle. The flat inner and outer surfaces of the shoulder blades are lined with muscles that attach to the sides of the ribs and to the upper arm inside the armpit. These muscles form a cuff that connects arm, shoulder, and rib cage, and determine "home base" for your shoulders and arms. Connecting this cuff to the lower torso is a broad V-shaped sheet of muscle that runs from the upper arm around the back of the rib cage, through the thick fascia of the lower back to the rim of the pelvis.

Ideally, each collarbone lies horizontally from the highest tip of your breastbone to the cuff of your shoulder, where it's connected by ligaments to the outside corner of your shoulder blade. The interface of collarbone and shoulder blade forms a shallow cup into which your upper arm fits. The shallowness of this socket allows for the extreme range of motion of the arm and also makes it susceptible to displacement. Your shoulders are the most structurally unstable part of your body, but that instability is exactly what lets your arms be so versatile and expressive.

The only place where the parts of your shoulders fit solidly together, bone on bone, is where the collarbone meets the breastbone. That connection is a pivot point around which the collarbones move. When the collarbones move forward, the shoulder blades and the tops of the arms roll forward too. Hollow indentations above and below the collarbone indicate that the collarbone is riding too far forward in relation to the rib cage.

For a variety of reasons—because our work causes us to look forward and down, because forward flexion of the body provides a feeling of security, because our breathing is restricted, or because flexion is an efficient spring for fast takeoffs—most of us have depressed rib cages, the result being that the breastbone cannot properly support the collarbone. As our collarbones roll forward, our shoulder blades wrap forward around the ribs like a stole. To maintain this posture, the muscles on the front of the shoulders and arms become chronically shortened, and the muscles that should connect the scapulae (shoulder blades) to the spine and pelvis become flimsy and passive. Consequently, the shoulder blades form "wings" that slide around disconnectedly, pulled along after the arms. In balanced shoulders, the scapulae stay behind on the back except at extreme ranges of motion. The shoulder blade is meant to function as the connecting link between the arm and spine.

Displacement of a shoulder blade may be masked if the rib cage is depressed and the upper spine is curved. Muscular bulk, especially in men, can cover a multitude of structural imbalances.

A "shoulders-back" stance only aggravates poor posture by adding the muscular tension of an inauthentic pose. By now you're familiar enough with how compensation works in the body to realize that just *putting* a body part where you think it belongs only results in some other part going awry. Forcing your shoulder girdle back means that some portion of your spine compensates by pitching forward. It may be your lower back, the area between your shoulder blades, or your neck. Try it and see. Competent use of your arms depends on balanced alignment of your shoulder girdle, which in turn depends on support from your rib cage, spine, pelvis, and legs.

Using this map of the shoulders, have your partner help you explore the actual terrain. Place your hand on your partner's shoulder blade and ask him to slowly move his arm around at random. Feel the relationship of the shoulder blade to the arm, and notice the adjustments the collarbone makes. How connected does the shoulder blade feel to the spine and rib cage? Does it feel welded on, or does it slide all over the place?

Now take some time to become aware of your own shoulder pattern. Act out some typical tasks that you perform every day—brushing your teeth, washing your hair, rinsing dishes. Notice how your shoulder blades participate in the action. Then sit down, and placing your arms on an imaginary steering wheel, mime the motions of driving. What are you doing with your chest, shoulders, and head? Notice how the movement feels, and imagine how it would look if you could step outside your body and watch. Make an imaginary video of yourself at the wheel to refer to later on.

Spine and Shoulder Blade Support for Your Arms

As preparation for the arm and shoulder explorations, please review script 4 in chapter 2 (page 34). This will remind you of your full-body breathing, your back and side dimensions, and the correspondence between the "umbrella" of your ribs, your respiratory diaphragm, and the floor of your pelvis. All dimensions of your torso are needed to support your shoulders.

Script 24 briefly reminds you of three-dimensional breathing. The new image of gills under your armpits evokes breadth across your shoulder girdle. Then, raising your arm toward the ceiling and finding a place of balance, you'll experience gravity's support for your arm.

You may have already done this exploration long ago when you were a kid. You were probably lying on your bed talking to your best friend on the phone, absentmindedly balancing one arm in the air. Or maybe you used to balance a broom handle in the palm of your hand. Most of us have forgotten those simple, pleasurable games with gravity. This script contrasts the feeling of using muscular effort to hold your arm up with the feeling of letting it be supported by your back and by gravity.

SCRIPT 24

EXPLORING SHOULDER SUPPORT

Lie on the floor, knees bent and feet close enough to your hips that your legs feel supported by your feet. Let your legs relax. Feel your breath as it deepens into the pause at the end of your exhalation. And notice your rib cage responding to your body's need for more air, . . . air coming in, . . . and air flowing out. You can feel the back of your body softening, . . . and yielding to the floor. And you can notice your upper ribs opening like an umbrella. This movement reverberates down through your diaphragm, . . . and down to your pelvic floor as you breathe in, . . . and out.

And you remember how your internal core flows lengthwise through your body, like a sheltered mountain stream, . . . flowing down through your legs, . . . into your feet. And branches of the core flow upward through your heart, . . . and out into your arms. As your shoulders soften, . . . you can feel the movement of your breathing under your armpits, widening your upper rib cage. Imagine that you are breathing in and out through gills under your armpits.

With your arms resting parallel to your torso, gradually bend your right elbow and draw your fingertips toward your shoulder. Move very slowly. As your fingertips approach your shoulder, your shoulder blade relaxes back, . . . yielding to the added weight of your forearm. And as you continue breathing, . . . you can feel your shoulder blade spreading out against the floor. And continue to let your shoulder blade settle as you raise your elbow toward the ceiling. Let your forearm and wrist stay passive. As your upper arm approaches vertical, you'll find a place where your arm settles in, . . . your elbow seems suspended in the air, . . . supported by gravity.

And now gradually unfold your elbow, extending your forearm toward the ceiling. Extend your wrist, so your fingers point upward. Let the weight of your whole arm settle down into your shoulder blade. You feel as though your arm could balance there for a long time.

Now, with your arm still suspended, contract the muscles in your armpit. Pretend you're trying to hide a coin in the crease. Notice the tension this causes in your shoulder, neck, and upper back. And now release that imaginary coin, letting your armpit soften. Feel your arm relaxing in its socket, . . . and notice how softness in your neck, back, and shoulders lets gravity support your arm.

In a moment you're going to let your arm drop back to its starting position alongside your torso. It will fall when you exhale. Keep your elbow and wrist straight but not locked. When you completely relax the muscles in your armpit, your arm will fall like a tree in the forest. Now breathing in, . . . exhale and let it fall.

Repeat this first part of the script for your left arm and then continue with the rest of the exploration.

Slowly raise your right arm to the vertical position. Relaxing your shoulder blade, . . . let your arm settle into the shoulder socket.

Now reach your fingertips toward the ceiling, so your rib cage and shoulder blade are pulled up off the floor. Notice how much effort that takes. Then, with an exhalation, let your ribs settle back into gravity. . . . Let your shoulder blade relax. And let the weight of your arm settle into your shoulder joint. Notice how much easier it is to relax and let gravity support your arm.

And, as you exhale, . . . let your arm fall like a tree.

Repeat this exploration for your left arm. If one arm has difficulty feeling gravity's support, spend more time with that side.

———————————◆———————————

Claiming Your Elbow Room

Most people support their arms with tension along the top of the shoulders and in the neck, relying on muscles of the upper arm for movement. This pattern makes the arms look and feel disconnected from the rest of the body. Once you can let the weight of your arms be supported by your shoulder blades and back, their movement will feel smoother and more connected.

All the muscles that determine balanced shoulder action attach to your upper arm—your forearm is not involved. A simple way to focus your attention on the movement of your shoulder is to pretend that your arm ends at the elbow.

Script 25 teaches you to guide your arm movements from your elbow. It also helps you relax the armpit area where your arm and shoulder blade can be bound too tightly. When your shoulder blade is free, it can mediate between your spine and arm and make the microadjustments necessary for smooth arm movement.

Remember to perform this exploration slowly enough to allow the subtle adjustments your body must make to connect your arms with your core.

———————————◆———————————

SCRIPT 25

GUIDING MOVEMENT FROM
YOUR ELBOW

Lying with your knees bent, let your body relax into the floor, . . . and let your breath flow through your core into your legs and feet. With your right arm bent, raise your elbow toward the ceiling, letting your fingertips dangle softly near your cheek. Feel your shoulder blade supporting the weight of your arm. In very slow motion, draw a small circle in the air with the tip of your elbow. Notice how your shoulder blade can softly adjust to the changing angle of your arm. . . . And now reverse the direction of your circle, still moving at a snail's pace.

Return your elbow to vertical. This time, gradually move your elbow sideways, away from your body. Breathing through your imaginary gills, . . . you can feel your armpit opening as your elbow approaches the floor.

With your upper arm now resting on the floor, you can feel your breath moving in your back, . . . between your shoulder blades. And slowly return your elbow to the vertical position, letting your armpit stay relaxed. As your elbow rises, your arm seems to be falling uphill, . . . and you feel the weight of your arm passing through the joint, . . . into your shoulder blade, . . . and into your back. . . . As you exhale, let your right arm return to a place of rest by your side.

Repeat the elbow circles and side extension with your left arm.

Now, with both elbows bent, fingertips at your neckline, raise your elbows toward the ceiling. And letting your breath expand the umbrella inside your rib cage, . . . move both elbows outward, away from each other. As your arms approach the floor, feel your upper back getting softer and broader, . . . and your armpits softening. Let your feet, spine, and rib cage settle deeply into the floor, connecting you to the earth.

And now, as you slowly raise your elbows back up toward the ceiling, . . . continue to let your spine give in to gravity. Let your lower body support the motion in your shoulder girdle.

Once your upper arms are vertical, extend your elbows so your wrists and elbows are straight but not locked. Let the weight of your arms settle into your back and shoulder blades. Now, with your legs and back supporting the movement, slowly move your straight arms apart from each other. Take five cycles of breathing for your arms to reach the floor. You can steer the movement with your elbows, even though your arms are extended. You have plenty of time to notice the dimension of your breathing, . . . and to feel your breath moving through the core of your body.

Let your arms hover just at the surface of the floor, so the core of your arms, shoulders, and back is active in this open gesture. Pause here for a moment to breathe through your imaginary gills. Then slowly raise

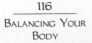

your arms to vertical, ... breathing, ... taking five inhalations and five exhalations. Your arms seem to fall upward, as their weight sinks into your shoulders and back. Place your attention on the path of your elbows, letting your forearms go along for the ride.

When you reach the top, pause for a moment. Then slowly repeat the arm extension to the side. Focus on the movement of your elbows and the supportive feeling in your back and legs. Let your throat and jaw stay relaxed. ... To finish, let your arms drop one at a time, like trees in a forest.

Notice the overall feeling in your body right now, especially in your shoulders, arms, and chest. Find some words to describe this feeling to yourself.

When you're ready, undo the feeling. Notice specifically what tensions you acquire. Do you tighten your neck or jaw? Does your breathing become more shallow? What about your armpits? your shoulder blades? your ribs? your thighs and buttocks? Once you've identified any old habits, re-establish the new feeling, noticing what steps you take to create it.

◆

The Arms Fall Uphill

In script 26, you'll raise your arm from beside your body to a flexed position, guiding the movement with your elbow and letting your shoulder blade accommodate to the shifting weight of your arm. You'll do this at moderate speed, training yourself to find home base for your arm without hesitation. Although you'll be lifting your arm, you'll have the sensation that your arm is falling uphill. This feels very different from anchoring the shoulder blade and lifting the arm against it.

You'll then practice the relaxation necessary to let your straight arm drop back down to your side without hesitation. If you have severe shoulder tension, you may find it strangely difficult to let your arm fall like a tall tree. You'll find yourself controlling your arm part of the way down, until it feels safe to let go. Or you may let your elbow bend instead of releasing only the muscles in your armpit. The goal is to focus the release in your shoulder joint and to let go all at once so your entire arm takes the plunge. One way to sort this out, if you have difficulty, is to lower your arm to an angle that feels safe for letting go. Focus on the free feeling of the moment when your arm is in flight. Take pleasure in that moment. Then gradually work up to a more vertical starting position.

◆

SCRIPT 26

ARM RAISE AND DROP

Lie on the floor with your knees bent, feeling support from the earth. Let your abdomen relax, . . . and be aware of breathing through your core. Your rib cage expands in all dimensions.

With your right arm lying alongside your torso, keep your elbow and wrist firm but not locked. Guiding your arm from the elbow, raise your arm toward the ceiling. Feel your back and shoulder blade giving in to the weight of your arm as it rises. Relaxing the muscles in your armpit, . . . let your arm rest into the shoulder joint, . . . and find a zone of balance. Your back and shoulder form the hull of a ship, . . . and your arm is its tall mast. Your arm could balance there, without effort, for a long time.

When you're ready, let your arm fall, all at once, back down to your side. Take pleasure in the moment when your arm is flying through the air.

Practice the lift and drop several times with each arm.

◆

Two Axles

Script 27 begins by helping you integrate the new balance of your shoulders with the balance of your hips and pelvis and to explore this integration in standing. You'll imagine a horizontal axle around which your arms pivot when they flex forward. With this axle in place you'll do the pelvic-roll motion, noticing the horizontal axle between your hips. When you roll up to standing, you'll become aware that your horizontal hinges are perpendicular to the vertical elongation of your internal core.

When you perform the pelvic roll, be aware of increased sensations of movement in your upper torso as you rotate your pelvis. The explorations in the previous chapters have relaxed your core so you can now feel subtle shifts of weight more acutely. When your core is open, the pelvic roll feels like a wave of energy passing all the way up into your head, a river flowing north through a canyon.

This script continues with a series of patterns that remind you of standing support; it then helps you explore arm movements in the upright position. The shoulder blade marries the movement of the elbow with support from the spine and pelvis. As this movement strategy becomes familiar, arm gestures are initiated from the underside of the arm rather than from the top of the shoulder and front of the arm. Balanced use of the muscles of shoulder and spine make the elbow feel weighted. This sensation of heaviness in the elbows helps repattern arm usage and release shoulder tension.

◆

SCRIPT 27

INTEGRATION OF SHOULDERS AND PELVIS

Lie on the floor with your knees bent, letting your feet and hips support the weight of your legs. Imagine a horizontal axis running through your shoulder girdle from armpit to armpit. This axle lies deep inside your rib cage and is perpendicular to your internal core. When you inhale through your imaginary gills, you can feel your shoulders widening across the horizontal axis.

Starting with your arms alongside your torso, raise them both toward the ceiling, guiding the movement with your elbows. Notice your arms pivoting around the axle, . . . and find the zone of balance when your arms reach the vertical.

Letting your arms rest there, imagine a second axis that passes through your pelvis from hip socket to hip socket. As you exhale, direct your sitting bones toward your heels and press lightly into the palms of your feet, ... letting your pelvic floor turn upward as your pelvis rolls back around its axle. Taking slightly more weight onto your feet, let your whole pelvis curl up from the floor. Notice how your weight rolls upward, ... flowing like a river through the canyon of your body, ... all the way up to your shoulders.

And slowly, let your weight return down through your core, ... through your pelvis, ... to rest. And let one arm drop, ... and then the other.

If your eyes have been closed, let them open now. Take a few moments to reorient yourself to your surroundings.

With a feeling of yielding to the earth, roll to the side and then onto your hands and feet. Position your knees about as far apart as your nipples. Push your weight onto your feet, but let your arms and body keep hanging down. Your neck can stay relaxed, and your head dangles upside down.

Remind yourself of your base of support in the palms of your feet, ... of the spaciousness in your pelvic floor, ... and the open feeling across the width of your pelvis. And still hanging upside down, remind yourself to breathe.

As you roll up to standing, your hinges work together, ... your ankles, knees, and hips unfolding, ... and your pelvis turning around the axle across your hips. As your spine comes up, your shoulders slide back around the axle across your shoulders. Your head continues hanging loosely as it rides upward on your spine. Your pelvic floor and diaphragm are spacious, supporting the weight of your torso. When your collarbone rises, your head comes up without effort, ... and rests on top of your rib cage.

Once you're standing, slowly bend your knees, taking one cycle of breath to go down and one more to rise. Centering your weight over the palms of your feet, ... slowly lower your pelvic floor about two inches. Keep your buttocks relaxed, letting your pelvis feel wide and open, as if you are sitting in a saddle. With your head erect, your eyes gaze softly forward. ... As you rise, you can feel the base of your support in the palms of your feet, ... and you're aware of the dimensions of your body, front, ... sides, ... and back, ... evenly distributed around your central core.

Standing easily, raise one arm forward from beside your torso to shoulder height. Relaxing your armpit and shoulder blade, ... imagine that your arm is being pushed up from below. Guide the movement

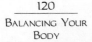

with your elbow. Feel your shoulder blade sliding along your back as it relays support from your lower spine to your arm. Breathing with your internal umbrella, let your upper arm find its home base in the shoulder socket. And then let your arm drop freely to your side.

Moving more quickly now, swing your arm up and down several times, letting your spine support the flexion of your shoulder. . . .

Explore this motion with your other arm. . . .

Now explore the motion with both arms together. Let your arms rise as you exhale. As your arms swing forward and up, feel your central core resting through the palms of your feet into the earth.

Letting your arms relax by your sides for a moment, place your right foot a step ahead of the left and begin rocking back and forth from the palm of one foot to the palm of the other. Keep your buttocks relaxed and your pelvic floor open, . . . letting the action of your legs reverberate up through your pelvis into your torso. Notice the natural swing of your arms that results. Keep rocking gently back and forth, . . . and gradually add a reach through your upper spine. Now your arms automatically swing higher. Let your elbows be guided up from the undersides of your arms.

And now use this motion as you imagine reaching for something on a high shelf. Pushing from your back foot to your front foot and simultaneously extending your upper spine, your arms reach up effortlessly.

◆

Handling the World

Take time to repattern some activities you usually perform sitting down. Sit at your workstation and run through some of your typical tasks. Remember the seated weight shift you explored in chapter 3? Initiate reaching movements of your arms by shifting your weight across the floor of your pelvis. Your chest stays open instead of collapsing, and by keeping its full dimension, it supports your shoulders. It also lets you breathe freely. As you reach across your desk for the phone, guide the movement with the underside of your elbow, letting your arm swing forward from your back.

In order to really get the hang of this, you must make sure your chair supports you properly. This is especially important for chairs in which you sit for long periods doing intense work. Ideal chair height positions your hips slightly higher than your knees, so the weight of your legs can be borne by your feet. Typical folding chairs and most tables and desks are suited for people who are about 5'7" tall. This means that the rest of us need to evaluate our workstations to make sure they fit our bodies.

Automobile seats are notoriously ill-fitting—their design is a combination of seductive cushiness and race-driver chic. Get some cushions to fill in those bucket seats and backs. And next time, buy a car with plenty of headroom, so you can be supported by your pelvis without wanting to cut a hole in the roof.

By the way, remember that video you made of yourself in the driver's seat? How does that compare with the way you're driving now? Remember to steer with your "heavy elbows."

Once you've got the knack of supported arm movement, try repatterning some familiar standing activities. Pick something simple and repetitive, like ironing a shirt or sweeping the floor. Remember to get support from your feet and keep your pelvic floor spacious. Let the heavy work be done in the lower part of your body, using your legs to shift your weight. Use your arms primarily for holding, guiding, or steering. Breathe freely, and let your elbows swing from your back. This will make vacuuming a whole new experience!

And check out your gait now. The added relaxation in your shoulders will make the movement of walking feel more connected all the way up your spine. Each footstep reverberates through your internal core.

The Gravity Gang

"It's all in the pelvis," Bill mutters to himself. He's determined to conquer his tennis serve. "Every time I screw up, it's that darn tail tucking under again. Makes me lose my ground."

He stops, gives his body a shake, and takes a few full, easy breaths, gazing out beyond the court to the children's playground. He watches some kids on the swings, unconsciously swaying his body from one foot to the other, matching their swinging motion.

"Okay," he says aloud. "My pelvis is supposed to be a relay station. If I tuck my tail under, it keeps the movement from going freely up my spine and out my arms."

He takes a few more practice swings, letting his pubic bone drop slightly and picturing himself with huge, hippopotamus haunches. It gives his legs more substance.

"Better," he thinks, "but something's still missing."

He hears the familiar "caw, caw" and watches a crow land on a telephone pole.

"That's it!" Now Bill flaps his arms up and down. Big black wings fan out from the small of his back to his elbows. He's oblivious to the spectacle he's making of himself. Stringbean no longer exists. As he swings his weight back over his right foot, his elbows fly into the air.

Whack!

"Killer serve!"

Pauline is lying on the living room floor with all four limbs poised in the air.

"You look like a dead bug," Margie teases, tweaking Pauline's big toe.

"Maybe," says Pauline, rolling over lazily. "But you know what? I think I finally understand what initiating movement from the core of the body feels like." She sits up, eager to share her insight.

"I really got it about letting my arms come out of my heart instead of being tacked on at the tips of my shoulders. It's like singing—it's got to come from *inside*."

"Tell me more," Margie says, sitting down on the couch.

"Well, I'm not using my arms that way all the time yet. But I sure do notice it when I'm not. Like at work. When that uptight feeling creeps over me and suddenly my shoulders are hiked up around my ears, I know I've let my core awareness slip away." Pauline pantomimes the attitude.

"What do you do when that happens?" Margie asks.

"Breathe!" Pauline swings her arms wide, breaking free of her imaginary straightjacket. "Remember that I'm a three-dimensional being. Then I remind myself to occupy my legs and let my pelvis open up so it can support my back. And, you know—those plates get so much lighter! And I'm wiping off tables guiding the movement with my elbow. It gets to be a game."

"Like, 'how can I do this job with the least effort'?"

"Right. Takes fewer muscles to smile than to frown, you know. And you know what else? I've decided to look for a better job. I'm starting to feel suffocated at the café. And I want to make more money. Maybe doing something like Fred does, in sales." Pauline sits down on the couch beside Margie.

"Sounds good to me," Margie smiles. "By the way, what's happening with Fred? You said he wasn't getting much out of the gravity explorations."

"Well, that's another story. I invited him to go to the ballet with me the other night."

"Not exactly his mug of ale, right?" Margie comments.

"He went though. And I got to wear my blue-sequined dress and silver heels. *That* was a cathartic experience. I've gotten so used to feeling connected to the earth these days, it was like walking on stilts."

"The price we pay for beauty, huh?"

"It was terrible. I started locking my knees again and that set off my lower-back pain. By the end of the evening even my neck felt tight."

"So what're you going to do with those silver sandals?"

"Wear them in my boudoir, I guess." Pauline laughs and strikes a provocative pose on the couch. "Oh, it wasn't really all *that* bad. We were sitting down most of the evening. But I sure wouldn't wear them out dancing."

"I'll bet. But you were telling me about Fred."

"Well, at intermission he started talking about the difference between the lead dancers and the corps de ballet. How the stars moved with less effort and more grace. That's what got me turned on to trying to find the core movement in my own body. The prima ballerina's arms were incredible, the way they seemed to flow out of her heart. But the corps dancers all looked like their arms were ordered from a catalog. They were good dancers and all, but they didn't look connected. It might seem subtle, but once you start seeing it, it isn't subtle at all."

"And Fred saw that?"

"He pointed it out to me! He's got a keen eye for movement. I just wish we could figure out the source of his back trouble. He's started getting chiropractic adjustments, and he says it helps. But he's agreed to give the gravity patterns one more go. I invited him over Sunday night to practice together."

"Hey, maybe I'll see if Bill can come too, if that's okay with you," Margie says. "He's been looking awfully smug lately. I won-

BALANCING YOUR
BODY

der what structural secrets he's discovered. Think about it and let me know. I have to get going now."

"Where to?"

"Sue asked me to see if I could help her with Matthew. He's only ten months old, and he already weighs twenty-two pounds. She's having a hard time carrying him around. Seems to me she's got to make some adjustment in her body to compensate for the extra weight of his body, but how to do it in a way that won't cause a problem in her back? It's sort of a puzzle."

"You really like this stuff, don't you?" Pauline observes. "Maybe you should be thinking about a new career too."

CHAPTER 7

HEADS AND TAILS

Just home from her Saturday morning singing class, Pauline hears what sounds like sobbing coming from Margie's room. Margie always has things so together—what can possibly be wrong?

Her roommate's door is ajar, so Pauline peeks in. Margie is curled up in a big overstuffed chair by the window, arms around her knees, her shoulders rocking gently. Tears stream down her face.

"Margie, what happened?"

Margie looks up, and to Pauline's surprise, smiles. Her face is soft and radiant despite red eyes and a mascara streak across her nose.

"Oh, Paulie, it's so amazing, this gravity work. I can't believe how deep it goes."

Pauline sits down on the rug near the big chair, hugging her own knees up to her chin. "What do you mean? You sounded so upset."

"Everything's fine, really," Margie says, straightening up and fluffing a cushion. "My universe just took a turn inside me, that's all."

"Now who's talking high drama," Pauline teases, relieved that nothing real has happened. She leans back on her hands.

But Margie's experience was real enough to her. "I'd just started the chapter on head balance," she explains. "The first thing you do is close your lips together tight and see if that tension goes anywhere else in your body. I was doing that when all of a sudden I felt like I was three years old. My grandma's yellow teapot is smashed to pieces on the floor. Mom and Dad are yelling at each other, and everything's all my fault."

Pauline notices how young Margie looks right now, like a little girl. "What was it like when you were growing up?" she asks.

"We were another 'dysfunctional' family, I guess. My dad worked hard at a humdrum job, came home and drank. Mom felt frustrated being a housewife but didn't know what else to do. She'd studied art in college but quit when she married my dad. They fought a lot, and Sue and I got caught in the middle."

Margie gets up and stretches out on her bed. Absentmindedly, she moves her toes and ankle up and down, watching her left foot as if it had a life of its own. After a while she continues talking.

"You know, I've sorted through all that childhood stuff in therapy—how I tried to be perfect to keep from getting blamed for everything. I've climbed the corporate ladder, and last summer I climbed a real mountain. I can see how my childhood motivated me to get where I am now. I like my life and where it's going. Really, Pauline, things are good. But today, for a few moments, I felt the strain of all the times I had to keep quiet so as not to disturb my dad, and the effort it took to keep my parents pacified."

Pauline nods sympathetically as Margie rolls over and rests her chin in her hands. "And it seemed like I've been doing that forever ... patching things up so other people won't be mad at each other. It all felt so tiring. It felt so good to cry and just go ahead and feel the way I did when I was little."

Pauline has been fascinated watching Margie's face change as she tells her story. When she talked about her dad's drinking habit, her jaw squared off like it did after a hard day at the office. But now her cheekbones seem wider and the edges of her jaw more round. Even her skin tone looks different, rosier.

The two women sit quietly for several minutes, each in her own thoughts. After a while Margie gets up and goes over to inspect herself in the mirror. She turns her head from one side to the other.

"What are your plans for today?" she asks at last, turning to Pauline.

"Nothing special. Thought I'd pick up some snacks for our get-together with Fred and Bill tomorrow."

"Would you have any time later on to read the scripts for me? I think I've let go of some tension in my head, but now I feel really spacey."

"Sure," Pauline says, privately marveling that Margie, "Ms. Self-sufficient," has asked her for help. "Maybe that book can help us figure out where your head belongs."

Getting Ahead of the Game

Tension in the neck, across the shoulders, and at the base of the skull is almost a given in our Western lifestyle. There are both structural and cultural reasons for this.

Spend fifteen minutes in a shopping center or on a busy plaza just watching people walk. Focus your attention on heads, those fifteen-or-so-pound weights we humans have to balance on top of our frames. Notice the quality of movement as people turn their heads to look at things or as they gesture with their heads in conversation. For the most part, you'll find these motions are abrupt and jerky.

Observe people's heads as they're walking along. Many people's torsos lag slightly behind their legs, so their heads jut forward to compensate for the imbalance below. Other people's heads and chests reach forward ahead of their legs. Either way, the head is not supported from beneath, and neck and shoulder muscles must tighten to keep it erect. This is the structural reason why necks become so rigid. A head that's free bobs subtly side to side or up and down depending on how a person's spine is responding to his gait. Most heads seem soldered to the spine like the knob on top of a flagpole.

What you rarely see is responsiveness, a head that floats along on the gait like a buoy on a lake. But then, most people have never been exposed to the experience of fluid support. Imagine fluid support flowing through a giraffe's neck in natural slow motion. Notice that movement of the lower body is reflected through the spine to the head. Right there at the very top, where the skull meets the first vertebra of the neck, is a slight give, a slight rocking motion as the head responds to the body's shift of weight. This is the location of the head's hinge.

If you watch some happy children on the go, you'll see the same thing. Their heads rock ever so slightly as they toddle across the lawn. Watch the children carefully, and you'll see that the movement takes place *inside* their heads, reminding you of those painted dolls from Chinatown with heads on springs.

The cranium actually does meet the first vertebra way up inside the skull, behind the soft palate and between the ears. Most of us move our heads from the base of the skull at the hairline and turn our whole necks in order to turn our heads. Our heads aren't free to move by themselves because the place where the movement should happen, up there between the ears, is the place where the knob is soldered to the flagpole. Movement at the core of the head and neck is inhibited by lack of support from below and by the resulting tension in the deep neck musculature.

At the other end of the spectrum from the children are the elderly. Some elderly people have their heads and necks so locked together that they must turn their whole bodies to look at something behind them. This is less a result of the aging process than of the chronic tension necessitated by structural imbalance. Structure, if addressed while it's still flexible, can remain flexible.

As a culture, we've learned to identify ourselves with our heads. We observe that those who get ahead have beautiful faces or clever minds, or both. Imitating them, we evaluate ourselves from the neck up. The body is something to be appeased, harnessed, and appropriately decorated to carry the head around.

Anthropologists discuss the religious origin of the split between mind and body in Western culture. Alternative medicine and psychology present approaches to healing that split. These approaches include consulting the body's wisdom. Rolfing Movement helps you integrate your head and body through physical support and balanced movement.

During your observation of heads and necks, you may notice how someone's counterintention is expressed in her structure. Maybe you'll notice a head jutting forward with a heart lagging behind, a common incongruity in our culture. Counterintention is braced with muscular stiffening, resulting in lack of responsiveness not just in the body but in the whole person; the split between mind and body results in a rigidified connection between the head and trunk. By releasing the head's grip on the body at the neck, old perspectives are often released as well. Congruent structure requires a flexible connection between the head and trunk. How reclaiming this flexibility affects feelings, attitudes, and behaviors is each individual's private adventure.

Tension in the face is another factor that causes the head hinge to freeze up. Tension at the jaw, under the tongue, and around the eyes and ears all affect the relationship of the head and neck. Our intentions and counterintentions are expressed in our faces as nowhere else in our bodies.

Masks of Tension

Script 28 begins by reminding you of the way the fascia throughout your body responds to the movement of your breath. You'll tune in once again to the gentle undulation of your core. You're then directed to interrupt your relaxation by closing your lips together as tightly as possible. This facial tension will produce rigidity in your throat and chest as well as a subtle tightening of the core of your body all the way down to your feet. By progressively relaxing the facial tension, letting go of it a little at a time, you'll be able to more keenly sense the connection between your face and body. If tightly pursing your lips is not a familiar facial expression, you can repeat the experiment with one that is.

People don't generally go around with the extreme facial tension that you'll experience in this exploration, but over time, any chronic facial attitude will take its toll on the freedom of the head hinge and on the fluidity of the structure below.

◆

SCRIPT 28

EXPLORING FACIAL TENSION

Lie comfortably on the floor with your knees on a cushion and your neck supported by a folded towel if desired. Let your attention follow the rhythm of your breathing, . . . the inhalation, . . . the exhalation, . . . and the pause. . . . You can feel your rib cage expanding, like an

umbrella opening slowly, ... feel your shoulder blades yielding as your
ribs open. As your diaphragm expands, ... the floor of your pelvis feels
the movement of your breath, ... and your whole body softens as you
exhale, ... and pause. As your legs settle lazily into the cushion, ... it
seems as if your knees are breathing, ... your calves are breathing,
... the soles of your feet are breathing. The core of your body resonates
to the rhythm of your breath.

In a moment you're going to do something that will briefly interrupt
the quiet feeling you have in your body right now. Remember that as
soon as you have experienced the interruption you can return to this
comfortable feeling.

Close your lips tightly together for several moments, noticing what
occurs in the rest of your body. Pay attention to the core of your body
as you press your lips together. Notice your breathing. Now, letting go
of half of the tension in your lips, notice what happens in the rest of
your body. And let go of fifty percent of the remaining tension in your
face, noticing how the core of your body responds, ... how your breathing responds. Continue reducing the tension in your face by half, keeping track of the changes in the rest of your body.

And letting go now of the last remnant of tension in your face,
... your breathing can resonate throughout your body again, ... and
your body is once more supported by gravity, ... safe at home.

◆

Releasing Fascia of
the Head and Face

Script 29 induces a deeply relaxed state to help you explore
your body image of your face. Since the face is familiar visually,
it may be a new experience to feel your face rather than see it, and
to sense the way your cranium supports your face. At the end of
the script, you're invited to undo the relaxation so you can become
more aware of your specific cranial and facial tensions. Then you
re-create the feeling of ease and openness.

SCRIPT 29

CRANIAL SUPPORT FOR YOUR FACE

Lie comfortably on the floor with your knees on a cushion, neck supported by a folded towel if desired. Let your breath gently open the umbrella within your rib cage. Notice the back of your head resting deeply into the floor, . . . the back of your cranium is a bowl into which your busy brain can settle, . . . and rest. And the bowl seems to have an elastic quality, so that as you breathe, the bowl widens, . . . and deepens, . . . opening more and more room in the back of your head. And your ears now seem to be floating on the rhythm of your breath, . . . floating ever so slightly apart from one another, making more room inside.

And now you imagine a little tube from each ear connecting inside your head, behind your nose, above your throat. And these ear tubes are elastic, . . . so you feel their gentle response to the rhythm of your breathing. You can follow a path from your inner ears down the back of your throat, . . . behind your Adam's apple, . . . down through your rib cage, . . . into a special, private place in your chest. And for a while you can enjoy sensing the connection between your head and this place in your heart.

And as you feel the inside of your head being supported by the elastic bowl of the cranium, you notice that your face can rest back into your cranium in a comfortable way. Your forehead feels smooth and wide and easy at the temples. And your lower jaw loosely hangs from your temples, . . . the roof of your mouth feels soft and wide. And with your lips gently together, you soften the space between your back molar teeth, and your lower jaw feels completely at rest. And as the root of your tongue relaxes, your tongue can be supported by the floor of your mouth. . . . Your eyes are soft and fluid as they rest deeply back into their sockets, . . . and the slight rocking motion of your breath, . . . makes your eyes feel like two small boats, rocking on the tide in a safe harbor.

The subtle motions you feel in your head right now echo all through your body. As you breathe in through your nose and feel the cool air behind your nostrils, you also feel a gentle pulse in the floor of your pelvis, . . . in your knees, . . . in the soles of your feet. . . . In a moment, you're going to undo this peaceful feeling and then re-create it.

Return now to the way your body felt before you began relaxing your face and head. Notice the familiar tensions that return to your head, face, throat, and upper chest. These tensions are like winter clothing you no longer need in the springtime. And now let these tensions dissolve as you re-create the easy feeling in your head, ... as your breath flows smoothly through the nooks and crannies in your head, face, jaw, throat, and whole body.

The Head Hinge

Rotation of the head, turning to the right and left, is possible because the top two vertebrae of the neck can function like a ball-and-socket hinge. Most people can't use this joint freely because of neck and jaw tension, so they overuse the surface muscles of the neck to turn the head. They rotate the whole flagpole instead of just turning the knob at the top. The first part of script 30 helps you rehabilitate the rotary motion of your head hinge. Remember to move in super slow motion—the less you do, the more you can feel at your core. The second part of the script deals with up-and-down motion of the head. Most people work too hard at this as well, raising the head by over-shortening the muscles at the nape of the neck and lowering by pulling the jaw toward the throat. In this script, you'll learn to guide the movement of nodding with the roof of your mouth instead of with your chin. This activates the horizontal axis between your ears, so the movement feels freer. With your cranial structure in balance, your neck and face muscles don't need to work so hard to move your head.

SCRIPT 30

PIVOTING AND NODDING AROUND THE HEAD HINGE

Lie comfortably on the floor with your knees on a cushion, neck supported by a folded towel if desired. Still remembering the fluid, responsive feeling in your head and face, ... your throat and chest, ... imagine a marker on the tip of your nose. Going slowly and smoothly, use the marker to circle the edge of a tiny dot in front of your nose. Spend two breath cycles drawing clockwise around that dot. ... And as you draw this small circle, let the weight of your face and head rest back into the bowl of your cranium. Your eyes rest softly in their sockets, and your jaw just rides along.

Now change directions and circle counterclockwise, ... noticing how the bowl of your head is gently rotating too. And it seems as though this movement takes place inside your head, ... way back behind your nose, ... and between your ears.

Next, slowly turn your head a few inches to the right, ... turning around the ball-and-socket joint inside your skull. Let the back of your head and hair slide against the floor, ... moving the back of your head to the left as your face turns to the right. And as you return the back of your head to its starting position, ... your face rides back to center, ... and the muscles of your neck stay soft, ... jaw and chin relaxed.

And, slowly turning the back of your head to the right, your face moves to the left. ... You can feel the motion taking place deep inside your head, ... and as you return to center, you can imagine the gentle motion at the core of your head echoing quietly down through the core of your body.

For contrast with this way of moving your head, slowly turn your head to the right and left in your usual manner. Notice the difference in the tension of the muscles at the nape of your neck, along your throat, in your jaw, and in the floor of your mouth.

Take a moment to restore the feeling of ease. ... With awareness of your breath, ... and guiding the motion with the back of your head, ... turn your head once more to the right, ... back to center, ... to the left, ... and back to center.

Continuing to breathe comfortably, ... allow your head to tip backward now, sliding the bowl of your cranium down along the floor. As you do this, the tip of your chin rises about an inch toward the ceiling. And now, as you exhale, ... slowly let the bowl slide back where it originally was, returning your face to center.

As you do this motion again, notice that when your head rolls back, the roof of your mouth moves away from your Adam's apple. With your head back, your throat feels open, ... the floor of your mouth is relaxed,

...the nape of your neck is relaxed,...eyes relaxed,...and you continue breathing comfortably. The weight of your head rests deeply into the floor.

To return your head to center, guide the roof of your mouth slowly down,...and let the muscles of your throat, lower jaw, and neck remain peaceful.

Imagine now a horizontal axis between your ears. Notice that this line is parallel to the axis across your shoulders,...to the horizontal dividers at your respiratory diaphragm and the floor of your pelvis, ...and parallel to the hinges at your hips, knees, and ankles.

And as you rock the bowl of your head backward once more, the roof of your mouth pivots upward around the horizontal axis between your ears. The movement is occurring deep inside, in the core of your head, ...your throat, neck, and lower jaw have nothing to do but ride along.

And now, letting the weight of your head settle back into the bowl, slowly let the roof of your mouth return to center.

For contrast, move your head up and down in a more familiar way. Notice what is happening at the nape of your neck, inside the top of your chest, and in your lower jaw and throat.

And now re-do the new movement. Remind yourself of the calm, open pathway that connects your inner ears with your heart,...and slowly let your head roll back around its axis,...and home again.

If your eyes have been closed, let them open now,...and reorient yourself to your surroundings. When you're ready, roll onto your hands and knees and unfold to standing as you have done in previous explorations.

♦

Approaching the World from the Back of Your Head

Script 31 explores movement of your head in the sitting position. When movement is balanced at the head hinge, the front and back of the head are equally weighted and the face feels supported by the cranium, even in the upright position. This balance also relieves eye tension. Most of us have little awareness of the backs of our heads, and our head motion is dictated by our response to what we are facing. Emphasis on the face distorts the muscular balance at the joint of neck and cranium. Script 31 draws your attention to the back half of your head.

After becoming aware of the back of the head sitting down, you'll get up and walk around for a few minutes. The back of your head does the traveling and your face just enjoys the ride.

Once you've completed script 31, go back and review script 23, Moving from Sitting to Standing, in chapter 5 (page 106). The relaxation of your jaw, neck, and shoulders will make your movement in and out of chairs surprisingly easier.

◆

SCRIPT 31

MOVING FROM THE BACK OF YOUR HEAD

Sit on a firm chair at the correct height for your structure. Distribute your weight over your tripod of support, and breathing easily, let your body rest into the open saddle of your pelvis.

With your eyes resting in their sockets, . . . gaze softly toward the horizon, letting your eyes receive what you see rather than reaching for it. . . . And now, become aware of the back of your head, . . . from your ears back around the bowl of your cranium. Let the back of your head have equal weight, . . . and equal importance, . . . to your face. And now, begin turning the back of your head to the right, . . . letting your face ride to the left. And you might imagine features on the back of your head, . . . eyes that look behind you, . . . and then let the back of your head slowly turn to the left, . . . letting your face go to the right, . . . imagining a nose there on the back of your head, . . . sniffing into the distance behind you.

Next, explore moving your head in various directions, . . . moving the back of your head up when you want to look down, . . . moving the back of your head back, . . . and letting the weight of your brain settle into your cranium, . . . as you gaze at the stars.

As you continue gently moving your head around, you can notice that the movement comes from the hinge way up inside, between your ears. And you sense support for the movement from the floor of your pelvis,... and from the palms of your feet, and from the earth. Feel how smooth that movement is. Compare it to the way you usually move as you look around.

Let your pelvis roll back to a more slouched position, the way you used to sit. Notice that this makes it harder to move your head in the new way. This is because you've lost your foundation.

Re-creating your support, once again move your head in a balanced way.

Review script 23, Moving from Sitting to Standing, now.

Once you're comfortable standing, walk around the room, letting your face rest on the back of your head, as your whole body moves forward together—head, heart, and gut in harmony.

———————————— ♦ ————————————

Structural Integration

Script 32 reviews several patterns introduced in the lessons on leg and shoulder hinges, integrates those motions with head balance, and guides you up to standing and walking. This script can be used as a general review of most of the Gravity Game patterns. It's a structural meditation, a movement mantra.

Once you've found support for your head in the standing position, you may have a sensation of feeling taller or shorter than usual. If your habitual pattern of tension has been to hold yourself up, the integrated relaxation process can make you feel closer to the ground. If your pattern is to hold yourself down or in, the new integration will make you look and feel taller and slimmer.

As you practice walking, have the intention of integrating fluid support through your whole body—all those smoothly oiled hinges interrelating with the grace and ease of an animal roaming free. With your neck and face relaxed, your head can respond to your gait like a buoy bobbing on a quiet lake. You might remember your body feeling like this long ago when you were a kid—so light and free you feel like dancing.

SCRIPT 32

MOVEMENT MANTRA

Lie with your knees bent, soles of your feet flat on the floor near your buttocks, feet and knees in line with your nipples. Let your breath circulate freely throughout your body, . . . feel your head and face responding to your breath, . . . and as your breath caresses the back of your throat, sense the response in the floor of your pelvis.

Slowly extend your right leg, sliding your foot down along the floor with your kneecap facing the ceiling. Let the weight of your leg settle into your heel and sitting bone. . . . Slowly flex your ankle hinge, letting your knee and hip passively bend with the movement. Now, relaxing your calf and foot, draw your knee upward toward the ceiling, letting your heel drag in toward your buttocks. As your knee arcs over your pelvis, your foot lifts from the floor, . . . and the weight of your thigh finds a resting place in your hip socket. When you're ready, relax the muscles at your groin, releasing your thigh, so your foot drops smoothly down onto the floor.

Notice any slight tensions that may have crept into your head and face while you were concentrating on the movement of your leg. Appreciate those tensions for trying to help you perform the leg motions perfectly. Remind yourself that you're learning to move your body with minimal effort. And let those tensions drift away, . . . knowing you can find them again if you ever really need them. . . . And as you tune in to your breathing again, you rediscover the open channel between your inner ears and your heart, . . . and you feel your jaw lazily floating on the tide of your breath.

Taking your time, repeat the patterns with your left leg—left leg sliding down, . . . ankle, knee, and hip hinges bending like a drawbridge rising, . . . leg gliding upward and over the pelvis, . . . releasing the groin, . . . and dropping the foot to the floor.

Directing your sitting bones toward your heels, lightly press both feet into the floor, . . . and with soft buttocks, . . . feel your pelvic floor turning toward the ceiling. . . . As your weight rolls back over your sacrum, . . . through the dimples at the back of your pelvis, . . . and on up through the middle layer of your rib cage, . . . your body responds all the way up into your throat and head.

Now, as you exhale, slowly reverse the movement, . . . letting your weight roll down through your core, . . . your lower spine lengthening, . . . your weight descending through your pelvis, . . . through your feet, and into gravity.

As your breathing ebbs and flows, . . . your arms seem to rock gently with the tide, like boats moored in a quiet dock. . . . Now, with your right wrist and elbow gently extended and guiding the movement with your elbow, . . . gradually raise your right arm to a vertical position. Let the weight of your arm settle comfortably into your shoulder joint, . . . supported by your shoulder blade, . . . and by your breath, as it expands your rib cage.

As you slowly raise your left arm, you notice that your arm can move without any help from your neck and jaw.

Letting both arms remain in the air, . . . and remembering the horizontal axis between your ears, . . . you smoothly roll your head back, letting the roof of your mouth tip upward, . . . resting the weight of your head into the bowl of your cranium. Then, with your jaw relaxed, . . . and your throat soft, . . . you let the roof of your mouth guide your head back down to a comfortable place, . . . opening a soft space at the nape of your neck. . . . And when you're ready, release the muscles in your armpits, and one at a time, let your arms drop back down to the floor.

If your eyes are closed, let them open now, and take the time you need to reorient yourself to your surroundings, . . . letting your body maintain a feeling of integration and wholeness. . . . Now, with a sense of giving in to gravity, roll to one side and then onto your hands and knees, . . . and push your weight onto your feet. With your head and torso hanging loosely forward, and staying centered over the palms of your feet, . . . gradually unfold the hinges of your legs. And when the axis across your pelvis has found its home, . . . begin to unfold your spine, . . . letting movement take place deep within the core of your body. And as your rib cage finds its full dimension, . . . and your collarbone rises, . . . you discover that your head is finding a new place of support, . . . just over your heart.

Let your eyes be soft as you gaze forward. . . . Now bend your knees slightly, letting your weight sink through the palms of your feet, . . . and with your pelvic floor spacious, . . . sitting bones and pubic bone released, . . . you slowly lower the floor of your pelvis about two inches. Breathing *comfortably, you can feel the levels of support in your body—pelvis over your feet, ... heart resting over your pelvis, ... and head resting over your heart. And the chain of support continues as you straighten your knees, ... reaching down through your feet and into the earth to rise.*

As you walk about the room, notice the fluidity of your hinges, ... the responsiveness of your whole body to each footstep. Your legs feel long, ... suspended from beneath your rib cage, ... as they swing down through your hip joints. ... Your thighs swing forward independently of your sitting bones, ... and your knees unfold effortlessly ... Each foot rolls from the heel through the palm, ... and across your toe hinge, ... cushioning your gait so the floor feels soft. With your spine, neck, and face relaxed, your head is massaged by your footsteps. You might remember your body feeling this way long ago, ... so integrated, ... so light and so free.

◆

The Gravity Gang

"And you remind yourself of the soft, open pathway that goes from between your ears, ... behind your throat, ... to a special place inside your chest. And breathing comfortably. . . ."

"Pauline, stop for a minute," Margie says. "I want to try something." She puts her hands over her ears. Pauline is puzzled but sits back and waits.

With her hands blocking out impressions of the external world, Margie can focus her attention down inside her body. A sensation in her chest feels familiar—familiar but not quite right. It's a tension in her breathing, a tight barrier right in the middle of her chest. As she focuses on the barrier, she notices something behind it. It feels like an old red brick. She has to breathe around the brick. But the brick is hollow, and inside it is pain. Not hers but her parents' pain. Tears fill the corners of her eyes.

Margie's jaw tightens for an instant, but then a deep breath fills her whole body, and the brick seems to dissolve. "It wasn't mine," she says aloud, the tears rolling down her cheeks. What wasn't? Pauline wants to know. But she doesn't ask, sensing that Margie needs some time to sort out her internal pictures. After a while Margie nods, and Pauline goes on reading.

When they've completed the scripts, Margie stretches and sits up. "Wow," she says, shaking her head and smiling enigmatically.

"What was going on?" Pauline asks.

It takes Margie a few minutes to find her words. "When I let go of my jaw," she says at last, "it seemed like a new world opened up inside my chest. It was scary, because I could see that it's an imperfect world, and there are lots of things in it I can't do anything about. This isn't news, exactly. I mean, I've come to the same realization before with my therapist. But now I feel like I understand it deep inside my cells."

"It's so incredible how much deeper your feelings go when you start exploring your body," Pauline murmurs.

"It gives me an idea . . ." Margie stares into space for a moment. "Something about timing. How our minds can understand things quickly but our emotions take longer, and our bodies . . . well, without some body awareness, we might never change at all!"

"So the mind is like lightning," Pauline muses, "the emotions like fire, and the body like . . . what?"

"Like clay—it's responsive once it's warmed up, and you can make any shape you want." Margie stands up and reaches her arms out wide. "Oh, it feels so good to have space inside me. I'm realizing that it's not how I position my chest that matters but how I occupy the space inside."

"It looks like you're standing taller too," Pauline observes.

In letting go of the tension in her jaw, Margie has also let go of an attitude of bracing for a fight, so her legs now feel comfortable a little closer together. With her legs right under her body she has better support. Pauline has learned a lot to be able to notice that.

As Margie tests her walking, Pauline notices a graceful, feminine quality emerging. She doesn't swagger anymore, Pauline thinks to herself.

Margie laughs. She's stopped walking to watch a movie going on inside her head. There's a loud crash, and she sees her three-year-old self stiffen as if about to cry. Just then Grandma scoops her up into her bosom. The screen door slams and her parents' angry voices fade with their footsteps down the sidewalk. "You're okay, little Margaret mine," croons Granny. There's a smell of roses, a taste of lemonade. "It was just an old yellow teapot," Grandma says, "just a tempest in an old teapot."

"What's happened to your roommate?" Fred asks. He gestures toward the kitchen where Margie is pulling a casserole out of the oven. "Has she fallen in love?"

"Sort of," Pauline replies. "Better ask her."

"Hey, Marge," calls Bill. "How come you're waxing so domestic? Get a date with that new VP?"

"Watch it," Margie says, setting a basket of chips down on the table. "Your tabloid mentality is showing. What you're seeing is a woman who is being structurally transformed."

"Well, something looks different. Tell us about it."

"I will sometime but not right now. The feelings are too new. I had a lot of insights while I was releasing some tension in my jaw."

"There was more to that chapter than meets the eye," comments Bill. "I've been wearing contact lenses for ten years, but I realize now that I still hold my head as if I had heavy glasses on my nose. Especially when I'm sitting at my desk." Suddenly Bill gets a familiar glint in his eye. "You know, getting a head is no mean feat."

"Bad pun, Bill," says Margie.

"Oh, give me a break," Pauline and Fred groan in unison.

"Speaking of eyes," says Fred, "it seemed like after I worked with the scripts my eyesight was sharper than usual."

"Something like that happened to me too," Margie says, "even though I have twenty-twenty vision. It makes me wonder if poor eyesight, and even poor hearing, are really inevitable consequences of getting older."

"Now that's something to think about," says Fred. "It makes sense when you picture all those stiff necks and stiff upper lips. How can nerves and blood vessels function normally in necks made of steel?"

"Before you two go off into your theories," Pauline breaks in, "I want to tell you about something that happened to me. I haven't done the head chapter myself, but I read the scripts for Margie. This is sort of embarrassing," she adds, as the group turns to listen.

"When I was in junior high there was this girl who had an adorable turned-up nose. She was blonde and popular, and I

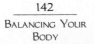

thought that if my nose were smaller, the boys would like me too. So I tried to scrunch up my face so my nose wouldn't stick out so much."

"Your nose is just fine," says Fred, touching its tip.

"I like it now myself," Pauline blushes, "but you know, I still feel that scrunched-up tension behind my cheekbones. And I'm thinking that if I can let it go, it might improve my singing even more."

"We'll sure give it a try," Margie says. "It's your turn tomorrow."

"This gravity stuff makes a lot of sense to me," says Fred. "You know, it would make a big difference if people could be more aware of structure when they start out learning things like karate or dance or even swimming. I still have a problem though. Even though my body feels more relaxed from doing these explorations, my back still gets cranky when I sit too long in one place."

"Walk around a bit, Fred," suggests Margie. "Maybe we'll get some insights if we can watch you move."

Fred paces back and forth across the living room, feeling slightly foolish. The others watch, trying not to let their usual image of Fred prevent them from seeing his structural pattern.

"Hear that?" asks Pauline. "He's syncopated. His right foot makes a heavier sound than his left."

"And look at his arms," says Bill. "The left one swings fine, but the right one hardly moves at all."

"Stand still," commands Margie, getting excited. "See, his whole right side looks lower than the left."

"You look like you're standing in a hole, old buddy."

"Bill," snaps Pauline. "Sometimes your humor is a bit much."

"It's all in the family," says Fred. "Just help me figure out how to dig my way out."

"Look," says Bill, holding up the book. "The next chapter is about balancing your right and left sides. Let's have dinner and then see what it says."

CHAPTER 8

SIDES
OF THE COIN

Mother Nature is no fan of symmetry. She likes balance but not visual symmetry. Symmetry requires immobility. Nature, on the contrary, is always on the move. The shape and angle of a tree and the whorls of its bark reveal the tree's interplay with the forces of nature. The varied and beautiful contours of the earth pictorialize its own slow-motion dance.

Humans seem to admire symmetry, cultivating static balance to pin things down. Within themselves, however, people are just as dynamic and asymmetrical as trees. From where do we derive this ideal of symmetry? Do we yearn for it because we don't embody it?

In considering human structure, symmetry is a useful concept as long as it's understood to be a guiding principle rather than an attainable goal. In the first place, the human form is obviously not symmetrical front to back or top to bottom. And a glance at an anatomy text reveals the asymmetry underneath the skin. So, were symmetry possible, the human form could approach it only on the surface, side to side.

Perhaps because there is so much duality on the surface of our bodies—two eyes, two ears, two arms, two legs—we expect to see symmetry when we look in a mirror and as we go through the day. But, especially on bad days, we don't. One eye is higher than the other, our smile is crooked, our shoulder bag slides off of a sloping shoulder, and we must have our pants altered to fit our shorter leg.

Noticing such things can be frustrating, until you realize that asymmetry is a message about a lack of dynamic balance. The shorter leg tells a story about imbalanced weight bearing and incongruent movement. The crooked smile indicates imbalanced tension in the jaw.

The concept of symmetry is a way of visually representing balance to ourselves. We can identify situations of imbalance or incongruence by contrasting them against an idealized picture of balance.

While left- or right-handedness is a factor in one-sided motions, most human movement is dictated by the two-sided design of the human structure. Human motion, like the flight of a bird, the growth of a tree, or the flow of geologic strata, is a dance with gravity. A harmonious dance depends on bilateral congruency, on being able to dance comfortably with yourself inside your own skin.

The two sides of your body don't have to look alike in order for this balance to occur, but they do have to communicate, to respond to each other, and to share responsibility. If one side consistently bears most of your weight and the other side is passive, your sense of center shifts toward the more active side of your structure. When your sense of center is displaced even a few millimeters, your body image becomes distorted. One side will feel fluent and flexible, the other side slow and stodgy. There may be disparity in the strength of the two sides or in the sense of competence.

When your body is in a balanced relationship to gravity, bilateral motions such as walking, cycling, and swimming feel congruent, with both sides doing an equal share of the work. Your body image on each side may not be identical, but the sides seem equally important, just as your front and back halves became equally important in the earlier chapters of this book. As you move, flexibility is matched with strength on both sides, work is matched with relaxation, and vitality is shared. When this is true, the visual appearance of your body comes closer to the ideal of symmetry.

Assessing Your
Bilateral Balance

Stand comfortably on both feet with your arms relaxed at your sides and your eyes gazing forward. Notice whether one foot seems to press into the floor more than the other. Do the knee-bend exercise (script 16, page 82), and notice whether one foot bears more weight when you reach the bent-knee position. When you straighten your knees, you may waver from side to side, relying more on one leg than the other to raise you up. It's hard to perceive this subtle preference at a normal pace, so go very, very slowly. If you were standing with your feet on two bathroom scales, which scale would register more weight?

Sit on a firm-seated chair with both feet on the ground. As you settle your torso into your pelvic basin, do you sense slightly more weight on one side of your pelvis? Is one sitting bone planted deeper into the chair than the other?

In walking, notice the sound of your footsteps. Does one foot land more emphatically? Do you spend more time on one foot than the other? Is the length of your stride longer on one side? How about the arc of your arm swings?

Awareness of disparity is an important first step. Yet, to force your body into a symmetrical movement pattern or shape would only add to your tension and cause you discomfort. The body image explorations in this chapter will aid you in developing an internal sense of harmony between the two sides of your body.

Taking Sides

The reasons for side-to-side structural imbalance are varied, but they always have to do with the body bearing more stress or activity on one side. This may be caused by repetitive one-sided movements or weight bearing, by injury to one side, or by unequal carriage in response to emotional association.

The body adapts its shape to the way it's used. The fascial webbing constantly orients itself to meet the pressures of stress and activity. But an imbalanced structural pattern that is repeated for many years becomes rigid and restricts the body's ability to respond to stress. A pattern that is at odds with gravity literally wears out, normally resulting in disability and pain.

Occupational imbalances are usually easy to rectify once you make a commitment to adjust the environment to your body. A carpenter might discover that his chronic low-back pain is aggravated by his heavy tool belt. Because he stows his tools on the side of his dominant hand, the belt throws his pelvis out of alignment. A solution might be to attach suspenders to the belt, so some of its weight can be born by his shoulders. He could also store the least-used tools on the nondominant side.

Anyone who must take notes while talking on the telephone will accumulate discomfort in the neck or shoulders. Cradling the receiver between ear and shoulder creates excessive tension in the neck. The tilt of the head puts extra weight on that side of the body, and this pressure can be reflected down the spine and into the pelvis. A simple solution is a lightweight headset, available through telephone accessory stores. It may be a slight nuisance, but it's better than using the neck like a hand to grip the phone.

Dentists do detailed work with their hands while bending across another person's body. Their left- or right-handedness tends to stabilize the spine in a predominant position. Add to this the mental stress of the consequences of some irreparable mistake. High-tech office equipment is some help, but these professionals also need to pay special attention to the way they use their bodies while working. Movement is the key—to change their own body position often, to move the client whenever possible, and to take frequent breaks in which they release their bodies from the static working position.

Repetitive recreational activities can be as detrimental to the body as repetitive work imbalances. A golfer's drive emphasizes a whole body twist from one side to the other. Years of this activity without care for the body will result in the twist being embedded in the fascia like creases in a dry streambed. A sudden movement against the grain is liable to cause injury. The golfer needs some activity that will soften this tension pattern. Slow yogalike stretching would help balance the flexibility of the two sides. Practicing a tennis backhand would help unwind the golfing drive.

One-sided body preferences can inadvertently be fostered in infancy. A child who is consistently carried on one hip develops a fascial tension pattern that accommodates to her mother's imbalance. Comfort and security become unconsciously associated with the resulting physical configuration.

As the child grows older, she may mimic or mirror a parent's physical attitudes. For example, if her mother has a habit of tilting her head to look at people when she talks to them, a child will mirror her mother's posture to achieve rapport. Looking sideways from the eyes is associated with astigmatic vision. Though the child's vision may be corrected with lenses, she may continue the habit of gazing sideways. This results in a rotated neck position as well as compensatory imbalance lower down in the spine.

Imbalance between the two sides of the body is also associated with a twisting curvature of the spine called scoliosis. A spine with scoliosis both rotates and sidebends, like a rope that, when twisted tightly, curves laterally. Most scoliosis is of unknown origin.

If you've been told by a physician that you have this curvature, pay special attention to your pelvis in the explorations in this chapter. Spinal curvature goes hand in hand with an uneven tightening of the deep muscles that thread through the pelvis connecting spine to legs. While severe scoliosis is rarely reversible, better balance in the core of the body and balanced support from the legs can help decompress the spinal curve and increase spinal mobility.

Traumatic Tension Patterns

Like repetitive usage or developmental patterns, physical or emotional trauma becomes embedded in the fascia, affecting the body's shape and mobility. The body reinforces itself around an insulted area to protect it from future trauma. This bracing is reflected throughout the body by way of the fascial network.

A traumatic tension pattern becomes an integral part of a person's body image. Strangely enough, the pattern is often so grafted to a person's sense of himself that he will actually be attracted to situations that are similar to the original insult. In so doing, he perpetuates the pattern by which he recognizes himself. The more he braces himself in his pattern, the less he can allow his body to be supported by gravity. By discovering the comfort of gravitational support, he can gradually release his internal bracing and expand his body image to include more versatile internal responses. As the fascia readjusts toward balanced functioning, the improved physical balance supports improved self-image and behavior.

Sometimes the habit of bracing can be corrected by simply practicing new patterns of bearing weight. Suppose someone broke her ankle years ago and ever since has protectively borne her weight on the outside edge of that foot. By learning appropriate

BALANCING YOUR
BODY

hinging of the ankle and foot, and integrating the new motion with the hinges higher up in her body, she can release the traumatic pattern. However, if there was strong emotion associated with the injury, she'll need to find a way to stop bracing against the emotional pain before the new physical pattern can be fully integrated. Processes to facilitate emotional restructuring will be introduced in this chapter and further discussed in chapter 9.

Body Symbology and Brain Hemispheres

Contemporary brain research tells us that the two hemispheres of the brain have distinctly different functions, the right brain being holistic and intuitive, the left brain logical and linear. Since each cerebral hemisphere controls the opposite side of the body, the left side of the body image tends to be associated with intuition, receptivity, creativity, feelings, emotions, and the feminine aspects of the personality. The right side of the body has to do with logical thinking, authority, assertive action, and the masculine aspects of character. Many people perceive these qualities as different types of energy in the body. Structural balancing can assist in the blending and integration of these energies.

A few people will find that the masculine/feminine relationship within the body is switched, with the more aggressive associations felt on the left and passive qualities on the right. Your own experiences and associations should always override any preordained pattern. Your personal experiences are what's real, and your individuality makes you interesting, the way a good cook's secret ingredient adds sparkle to a recipe. What matters in the end is how the flavors mingle.

Processing Emotional Associations

By seeking to organize your structure around the gravitational line, you are returning to a path of simplicity in your body. To stay on this path, you must let complications fall away. Complications include inefficient ways of moving, unsupportive environments, emotional baggage, or mental barriers. While the Gravity Game is based on awareness of structure and is primarily concerned with releasing and balancing patterns of physical tension, these patterns are intimately connected with attitudes, emotions, and memories. As you work on your body with the tools provided—awareness of internal body sensation, movement with minimal effort, and visualization—you may find that hidden emotions or forgotten memories are aroused.

The explorations in this chapter introduce processes to help you sort out any emotional associations that may arise as you work with your right/left balance. You can also use them to intensify your review of scripts from previous chapters. If you aren't aware of any emotional associations, read these scripts anyway; you may benefit from them unconsciously.

The processes in these explorations are derived from Neuro Linguistic Programming, from Arnold Mindell's Dreambody work, and from Eugene Gendlin's Focusing work. These body/mind approaches will be discussed in chapter 9.

Be sensitive as you work with this material. Self-help can go a long way, but sometimes emotional implications may be intense enough that you need the protection of an experienced witness. The appendix lists several body/mind-oriented and structural bodywork institutes that can refer you to a practitioner. Helpful books about various approaches to personal processing are listed in the bibliography.

It sometimes seems as though your tensions have a mind of their own, especially when you're trying to shed them. Always approach the Gravity Game with the attitude that your tensions mean well toward you. They've become embedded in your body to support you in one of two ways—to protect you from harm or to motivate you to some positive action. While you may not appreciate the discomfort that results from your tension, you can acknowledge its original good intent. The body seems to appreciate this mental attitude, and the more you cultivate it, the more your tensions will tend to cooperate with your desire to change. By the same token, there's no more certain way to get a tension to persist than to disparagingly chase it away. Try telling your shoulders they don't need to be tense after a long, hard day. You can almost hear them shout back, "What do you mean? We do too!"

In the following explorations, you'll learn to thank your tensions for their hard work and to enlist their help in finding new and better ways to support you.

You're evolving a new relationship to gravity through releasing, rebalancing, and integrating. This is a tall order to fill when you realize that your tensions have developed over the course of your lifetime. Change will probably occur in small steps. Appreciate the incremental shifts that indicate your body and self-image are changing. And be patient. It's okay for this process to take time.

The Gravity Gang

"Sounds like we're approaching ground zero," Bill comments, putting down the book. The four friends have decided to study right/left balancing together and have been taking turns reading.

"A little scary, huh Bill?" asks Pauline, squeezing in beside him on the couch. She grins at him mischievously.

"I don't know about that," Bill says, shrugging his shoulders and shifting his weight. "But I've been following all this brain research, and I think that since Western culture has become so materialistic and left-brained, and if the body hooks up to the opposite side of the head, then probably most Westerners' bodies are more tense on the . . ."

"Hey, Bill," Margie interrupts. Standing with her hands on her hips, she's shifting her weight from one leg to the other. "It sounds interesting. But could we save the conjectures for later, after we experience this stuff for ourselves?"

Bill feels a familiar knot tighten inside his chest. "Okay," he says, sinking deeper into the couch and stretching out one leg on the coffee table. "You're the boss."

"Thanks." Margie smiles, then turns to watch Fred. With a puzzled look on his face, Fred has been pacing the floor during the conversation, stopping every so often to bend and straighten his knees. "Have you noticed anything more about your bilateral balance, Fred?"

"Heavy on the right side, that's for sure."

"Anybody else discover they rely on one side?" asks Margie. "I'm right-sided too, it seems, though I never noticed it until now.

I sprained my left ankle badly when I was twelve, but I shouldn't think that would make such a difference."

"I never thought about my samples case either," Fred remarks. "In my last job I sold plumbing supplies, and I always carried the case in my right hand."

"Maybe you should have used one of those portable carts," Pauline offers, "like flight attendants use."

"It only weighed about thirty pounds," Fred says. "And in those days I'd have been embarrassed to use a cart. You know, 'real men' don't use carts! But I wonder why I didn't at least switch hands once in a while."

"We never think about these things," Margie says. "I'm glad I'm learning ways to help my nephew develop good habits right from the start."

"By the way, what ever happened with your sister's back pain? Did you figure out what was causing it?" Pauline asks.

"Sue was leaning back to counterbalance Matt's weight. It was as simple as that. I showed her how to find support from her legs and suggested she do some arm strengthening exercises to keep up with him as he grows heavier. But now I'm thinking about the habit she has of propping him on her left hip while she does things in the kitchen. I can't wait to figure out how she can keep him close and still get dinner ready."

"A maid," Bill says. "That's the solution."

"Maybe so," says Margie. "But I like the challenge. Let's go on with the explorations—maybe they'll give me some inspiration."

"Let's do it," Bill says. The sensation in his chest is quieter now, but he feels restless, even bored. He's not sure he likes working in a group like this but it would be rude to leave. He resigns himself to staying. "I'll read."

Scripts for Bilateral Balancing

Just as we assume that our bodies will appear symmetrical when we look in a mirror, we assume, major accidents aside, that our bodies feel symmetrical. Back when you practiced the fascial breathing exploration in chapter 2, you may have been surprised to find that the two sides of your body didn't feel the same.

Attending to those subtle sensations, you might have had the impression that the cells in various parts of your body were configured differently.

Return to script 3 now (page 31) and review that exploration, noticing any differing sensations in your two sides. Then go immediately to script 33, which will assist you in evoking balance between the two sides of your body image. The script suggests a way to let your nervous system blend the differing sensations. In this process you allow your mind to affect the substance of your body.

As you begin the blending process, you may experience some resistance. Perhaps your mind will wander or you'll become bored or anxious or feel some physical discomfort. Remember that your tensions have good intentions, so if your body resists merging the two sides, there must be a good reason. Scripts 34, 35, and 36 offer various processes for getting in touch with your resistance. Experiment to discover the approach that suits you best.

Script 34 suggests that you appreciate your resistance. Sometimes just acknowledging a tension will lead to a physical release. Script 35 suggests that you let your tension intensify. By focusing your attention on it in this way, you embrace it as an important aspect of yourself. Your intense focus on the physical sensation can result in a spontaneous shift from a kinesthetic to a visual mode of perception. In other words, the feeling can turn into a picture. This picture will have inherent meaning, like an image in a dream, and may lead you to an insight about the purpose of your tension. When you return your attention to the physical sensation, you'll probably find that it has changed, lessened, or even disappeared.

Script 36 is a shotgun approach for decoding the messages in your fascia. The questions in this script are designed to be gentle probes to assist you in releasing a tension and in understanding its positive intent. If you've been working with a partner, her familiarity with you and your body may give her a basis for intuiting which questions to read. If you're working with a tape, simply switch off your machine when you sense your body responding to one of the questions. You don't need to go through the entire list. One or two questions will be enough for any one session. And the list merely offers examples—tailor-made questions of your own may occur to you spontaneously.

A tension may disappear completely or it may lessen only a little during any one session. Respect the pace at which your body accepts change. When you've felt a release of tension through working with scripts 33–36, go on to script 37, which integrates the release with the supportive movement patterns you've previously learned. Script 37 also includes a slow-motion walking exercise that helps you alternate support between your two sides. The integration patterns insure structural support for your internal changes.

Sometimes, as you walk around exploring your new integration, you may find a resistance that asserts itself while you're moving. Maybe you'll feel an old familiar tightness across your chest, a tension in your jaw, or a foot that turns pigeon-toed. Again, go back to the techniques in scripts 34–36 to get in touch with the good intention behind your resistance. By appreciating the concern expressed by the tension in your jaw or exaggerating your toed-in foot as you continue to walk around, such patterns may spontaneously release.

After you've explored your new bilateral balance in walking, spend some time experimenting with other everyday activities such as working at your desk, doing household chores, or practicing fitness routines. Now that you're more aware of this aspect of structural balance, you may be surprised to discover how much you rely on one side of your body. To the degree that you continue your old pattern, you reinforce your bilateral imbalance. In an intense activity like weight training, this can be a significant influence on your structure.

◆

SCRIPT 33

BLENDING QUALITIES OF YOUR PATTERN

Review the fascial breathing exploration (script 3, page 31) before moving on to this script.

Script 3 has taken you on a journey into the interior of your body, where you may have noticed some differences in the way you experience various parts and regions. Perhaps the quality of one whole side is different from that of the other. Or maybe one thigh feels different from the other, . . . or one hip, . . . or one side of your chest, . . . or one shoulder. Wherever the disparity is most noticeable, focus your attention there.

Let your mind play with your sensations. If the two sides of your body were different colors, how would they look? . . . If the two sides had different sounds, what would you hear? . . . Do they have different shapes, . . . textures, . . . weight, . . . energy?

You can appreciate the special qualities of each side. Perhaps you appreciate one side for its strength and the other side for its gentleness, . . . or you might appreciate the smoothness of one side and the alertness of the other. . . . Spend some time now feeling and appreciating. . . .

After letting each side know that it is valued, . . . explain to your body that you wish to extend its choices to include all the variations between the two extremes. Neither quality will be lost, but both will be enriched. And you can ask the creative part of yourself for help, . . . let your creative self begin to merge and mingle the two qualities. You might imagine yourself cooking a special soup, adding a few seasonings from one side, . . . and then the other, . . . then returning for more of the qualities from the first side, . . . and from the second, . . . making just the right blend of tastes, . . . textures, . . . colors, . . . or sounds. You can be doing this unconsciously while you rest in a dreamlike state, . . . trusting your wise, creative self to do whatever is appropriate. Take all the time you need.

And when a subtle shift has taken place in your body, you will recognize it. Perhaps you will see your colors blended. Perhaps you will hear a new sound, . . . or sense that your breath now moves freely through both sides of your body. Notice whether the new feeling in your body is comfortable, . . . pleasurable, . . . whether it feels like a relief, . . . or whether there is some part of you that objects to the new blend, . . . that might prefer to let your two sides stay separated.

If the new feeling is acceptable to you, go on to script 37. If you feel resistance to the merging process, go on to script 34, 35, or 36.

SCRIPT 34

APPRECIATING YOUR PATTERN

Perhaps you feel a tense place in your body, a place that feels sepa-rate from the rest. You might sense it as a barrier between the right and left sides, . . . or you might feel it as a place where the movement of your breath does not flow freely. Perhaps your breath has to travel around that place to get where it is going.

Focus your attention right there, . . . and with curiosity, . . . and compassion, . . . go inside that place. You can appreciate its separateness, . . . its individual nature, . . . and even though the tension may feel uncomfortable at the moment, you can acknowledge it for its positive intention, . . . even though you may not yet know what that intention is.

Perhaps your body feels like moving a little bit, . . . gently moving around the area of your resistance, . . . getting a better sense of how the protected place really feels. As you experiment with tiny movements, you can notice what feels good, . . . and what feels uncomfortable.

And perhaps now, without knowing why, you notice that the tension has softened a little, . . . a shift has occurred inside, . . . and the separate place no longer feels so separate. . . . Your breath can pass through freely now, . . . and sensations from your two sides can blend. . . . Let your body tell you if this shift has made a difference, all the difference it needs for now. And if your body feels satisfied with this shift, you can draw your knees up, and with the guidance of script 37, begin to integrate this feeling with the movement patterns you've learned before.

If the resistance you have been focusing on seems to need more attention, scripts 35 and 36 offer additional ways of working. It is also possible that your release of that tension may lead you to discover resistance elsewhere in your body. Should that happen, you can repeat this exploration focusing on the newly expressing tension or work with it using script 35 or 36.

SCRIPT 35

EXAGGERATING A TENSION

Remind yourself again of the comfortable feeling of letting gravity support your body, . . . knees resting comfortably on your cushion, . . . thighs and buttocks peaceful, . . . your lower back cradled by the mat, . . . your abdomen resting back into your pelvis. Feel your rib cage gently expanding in all directions, . . . your heart resting within your rib cage, . . . and your brain settling into the bowl of your cranium. And let this sense of support remain with you, in the background of your awareness, . . . a safe place that you can return to whenever you wish.

And now, turning your attention toward the resistance in your body, . . . the place where your breath takes a detour, . . . you decide to experiment and let the barrier become bigger, . . . as if you were looking at it through a magnifying glass. And as you courageously exaggerate that feeling, . . . you may discover that the feeling spontaneously turns into a picture, . . . some image or scene that seems familiar or somehow meaningful to you.

As you watch the image, it might begin to shift and change, . . . perhaps even accompanied by sounds or voices. And this image may be bringing you some message, . . . something important you need to know to become more comfortable within yourself. . . . And still breathing peacefully, . . . remembering that you are supported by gravity, . . . allow that message to be stored away in a safe place, where you can find it again if you need it.

And as you appreciate this new information about yourself, . . . you may notice that the resistance in your body feels different: . . . perhaps it has become permeable, . . . perhaps its edges have softened. And you can appreciate the comfort this difference makes in your body. . . . And drawing your knees up, you prepare to integrate this difference into your overall movement pattern.

Go to script 37.

◆

SCRIPT 36

ELICITING MESSAGES

Perhaps the separate place in your body is a shy place, . . . perhaps it does not know the best way to communicate with you. In a few moments, you'll hear some questions that will help your body respond. Some of the questions will be meaningful and evocative for you, others will not. While listening, continue to focus on that special place in your body, letting the questions be directed to it rather than to your mind. When you sense that your body is answering one of the questions, turn off your tape or signal your partner to pause. When the tension has responded, go on to the integration patterns (script 37).

Remembering the way your body feels when it completely trusts the support of gravity, . . . and continuing to breathe comfortably, . . . you might ask yourself:

"What is in the center of this resistance? . . ."

"Does this separate place in my body keep something in, . . . or keep something out? . . ."

"What would my body feel like if the barrier were not there? . . ."

"Is there something that could happen somewhere else in my body that might let the edges of this barrier soften? . . ."

"If I could take this tension outside of my body and hold it in my hands, how would it feel? . . . If it had temperature, would it be colder or warmer? . . . How much would it weigh? . . . What would be its shape, . . . its color? . . ."

"If my tension turned into sound, what would I hear? . . ."

And you might address your resistance directly:

"What is your intention for me? . . . Is there another way that we might achieve this intention together? . . ."

"Do you have a message for me? . . ."

"Is there something you want to show me about myself? . . ."

"Is there something I can do to make you feel better? . . ."

"What keeps you feeling separate from the rest of me? . . ."

Once you have received an insight from your body and have felt your tension soften, let your attention gradually return from your inward journey. Feel the air against the surface of your skin. Sense your body's weight supported by the floor. Become aware of sounds in the room and of light filtering through your eyelids. Let your eyes open and notice your surroundings. Respond to your body's need to stretch or move about in any way. When you are ready, move on to script 37 to integrate the release of your tension.

◆

INTEGRATING BILATERAL BALANCE

You're now invited to incorporate your new relationship between right and left into your feeling of being supported by gravity. The new sense of balance will make a difference in your experience of the following familiar movement patterns.

Lying with your knees bent, knees supported by your feet, sense your breath flowing easily through the core of your body, . . . from your head, resting comfortably back in the cranial bowl, . . . through your shoulders and arms, . . . through your rib cage, . . . and through the floor of your pelvis, . . . all the way down to the soles of your feet.

Slowly slide your right leg down along the floor until your knee is extended. Then, letting the weight of your leg rest into your heel and sitting bone, flex your ankle, allowing your knee and hip to bend. Slowly draw your knee toward the ceiling, relaxing your calf and foot. As your heel drags up toward your buttock, your foot rises from the floor and your knee arcs over your pelvis. Pause, letting the weight of your thigh rest into the hip socket. When you're ready, relax your groin muscles and let your foot drop freely back to the floor.

Repeat this pattern on the left side, slowly extending your leg, . . . flexing the hinges, . . . dragging the leg upward, . . . arcing over the pelvis, . . . resting your thigh in the hip socket, . . . then release and drop.

Pause now to let your wise, creative self continue to deepen the communication between the two sides of your body. Spend a moment breathing comfortably and sensing the merging process.

Enjoying the feeling of integration, let your sitting bones ease down toward your heels as you lightly press both feet into the floor. . . . And as you exhale, allow your pelvic floor to turn toward the ceiling, . . . and your weight to roll upward through the back of your pelvic basin. Continue the movement, letting your weight travel uphill through the back of your body toward your shoulders. . . . And now slowly reverse the motion, unfolding your spine, . . . rolling your weight down through your sacrum, . . . and releasing your weight into your feet.

Starting with your arms relaxed by your sides, wrists and elbows extended, . . . and guiding the movement with your elbows, . . . let both arms rise to a vertical position. Your neck remains at ease, and your throat stays soft to let your breath through. Let the weight of your arms settle comfortably into your shoulder blades, supported by your back and by gravity.

When you're ready, release the muscles in your right armpit, and let your right arm drop. . . . Now release the muscles in your left armpit, and let your left arm drop.

If you've been working with your eyes closed, you can now become aware of the light through your eyelids, . . . and let them gently open. Still aware of being supported by gravity, begin noticing your surroundings, . . . the shapes and colors in the room, . . . and the sounds outside.

Once you have returned to the present, roll in a relaxed manner onto your hands and knees. Sensing the full dimension of your body, . . . and centering your weight equally between both feet, . . . gradually unfold yourself to a standing position. Notice how little effort is required as you smoothly rise through the core of your body.

Take a few moments to get your bearings in the upright position. Gently settle into the palms of your feet, letting each leg have an equal share of your weight. Now slowly bend your knees, settling down into the wide internal saddle of your pelvis.

Remembering to breathe, you rise by reaching down through the palms of your feet. As you slowly come up, you may notice that your weight wavers slightly, . . . that one leg feels stronger or more confident than the other. And you can thank that side for working so hard to support you. Let it know that its strength is valued, and that you would like to share that strength with other parts of your body. Ask your less confident leg if it would be willing to assume some of that strength, to accept just a little more of your weight than usual. And you can allow the two sides of your body to continue their dialogue in this manner, . . . while you slowly repeat the knee-bend pattern two more times, all the while remembering to breathe.

And when you're ready to explore walking, be gentle with the emerging feeling of balance between your two sides. Go very slowly at first. Start with your left foot a short pace ahead of your right, with the majority of your body weight balanced over the palm of your right foot. Gradually let your weight flow across to the left side, letting your leg and foot hinges be responsive, . . . until your weight is centered over the palm of your left foot. . . . Now let your right leg swing down through your pelvis and take a small step ahead of your left. . . . Then let the weight from your left side blend into the right until the weight centers over your right foot.

And repeat this process, letting your left leg swing down and forward, . . . and as your weight flows into the left foot, acknowledge your left side for its willingness to support you. . . . Then swing your right leg down through your pelvis and move forward again, allowing your weight to be fluid, . . . appreciating the special way that your right leg supports you.

Gradually assume a normal pace and length of stride as you walk around the room exploring the emerging harmony between your two sides.

<hr>

The Gravity Gang

Fred has been noticing that his right side feels denser than his left, as if his cells were packed more closely together. The left side is almost hollow by comparison. Seeking the source of the density, he notices a sort of vibration in his right knee. When he was fifteen, he'd torn some cartilage in his knee in a skiing accident. It'd seemed like no big deal at the time. He underwent routine surgery, and with the help of some good physical therapy, he was back on the slopes the following winter.

Maybe I unconsciously guard that knee, he thinks. Well okay, knee, thanks for being careful.

At this point, Fred notices that the heaviness in his leg has shifted somewhat, but it hasn't gone away. In fact, curiously, it feels a little worse.

I want to track this down, he thinks. I'm tired of feeling off-balance. He decides to intensify the sensation in his knee. It becomes very dense, like a steel ball bearing—a steelie—the kind he used to use to beat Bruce at marbles. Suddenly Fred feels a choking sensation in his throat. He coughs and sits up, staring into space. In a moment he rises and leaves the room.

"Are you alright, Fred?" Bill calls after him.

"You bet. Just go on without me."

Outside on the porch steps, Fred looks back into the past: it had been tough having a retarded older brother. Fred had covered up his embarrassment by ganging up with his pals and being mean to Bruce. Looking back, he feels ashamed. He takes a deep breath and sighs. Bruce is thirty-eight now and lives in a home for retarded adults. "Guess I've been storing my guilty feelings about Bruce down there with that old skiing injury. Strange, but that's how it feels." He remembers the last time he paid Bruce a visit, way back last fall. Too long ago, he thinks. He sees his brother's odd, rolling gait, the clumsy ceramic pots he had so proudly displayed, and the love in his brother's pale eyes. Fred puts his head in his hands and lets his tears flow.

At length, Fred sighs again, noticing how bright the stars seem all of a sudden and how soothingly the night air touches his skin.

Margie, meanwhile, is having her own adventure. The right side of her body is red and the left side a muted turquoise. She decides to twirl the colors together like cotton candy, and then the candy turns into a rainbow that seems to flow all through her body. These images make no sense, she thinks, but it's a pretty trip.

As Bill reads the part of the script that asks whether any part of the body objects to the new blend, Margie feels a cramping sensation in her left foot. It's a familiar pain that sometimes bothers her in the middle of the night. It's odd too, because that foot never hurts her when she's running. Scanning her body image again, Margie notices that the rainbow colors are sparkling everywhere except in her left foot. Down there the colors are vague and brownish. "I know you're trying to do something for me by being that way," she says to her foot, "but I can't think what." Margie breathes, letting the swirling colors bathe the inside of her body. "Or maybe there's something I could do for you. What would that be?"

Now there's music in her head—an old sixties song. She can hear the melody but can't remember the words. Maybe it doesn't matter. What grabs her attention now is a tingling in her foot. Looking down inside her body she sees the rainbow crossing the barrier at her ankle. "Now we're not going to discover a pot of gold down there, are we? That would be too much."

Since there's no response to her last question, Margie turns her attention to the gravity integration patterns. These simple movements have begun to seem like old friends, and it's pleasant to notice the subtle changes in the way her body responds to them. The whole left side of her body feels more alive, all the way up to her shoulder.

Fred returns to the group just as Bill is reading, "And you might ask your barrier if it has a special message for you."

A message, Fred thinks, stretching out on the rug, yes, I think there's a message. . . . As he closes his eyes, he sees Bruce smiling at him. And then the two of them are walking, Bruce leading him toward a building in a strange neighborhood. The sign on the building has special meaning for Fred. "Okay, I'll do it," he mutters, concentrating on a tickling sensation that's traveling up the right side of his body. As Bill reads the integration patterns, Fred notices immediately that the balance between his legs is different. Since he's not gripping the muscles around his right knee and hip, he can let his weight be more evenly distributed. And this makes his back feel better. With an uncanny feeling, Fred mutters, "Thanks, Bruce."

"How was that exploration for you, Fred?" Margie asks when they've finished reviewing the integration patterns. "You seemed to be going through some changes. And your walk sure looks different."

"It feels different too. I remembered some stuff about an old knee injury."

Margie starts to inquire but Fred is already moving past her. He'll tell his story when he's ready.

"What's that I'm smelling?" Bill calls to Pauline, who had disappeared into the kitchen midway through the scripts.

"Just a quick banana cake. I figured we might like some dessert after all this work."

"Pauline, what happened?" Margie asks, moving toward her friend. "I thought you wanted to do the explorations."

"Well, I bumped into something I couldn't understand," Pauline says. "Maybe you can work with me on it some other time. It felt like a big, dark hole. I couldn't appreciate it, and I was too scared to intensify it. Seemed like the best thing to do was put a cake in the oven."

"I'm sorry. I thought working together as a group would be a good idea," Margie says, putting her arm around Pauline's shoulder.

"It's not a bad idea. I'm learning a lot by watching the rest of you. Sometimes I think I can actually see your bodies changing as you do the inner dialogues. When a tension releases, it looks kind of like a candle melting in the sun."

"You don't mind then."

"Not a bit. I'll have dessert ready in a minute. Then I want to hear about the changes you were feeling."

Back in the living room, Bill is holding forth again. " . . . the impact of left-brained cultural norms on human structure. Think about it, Fred. Take some native Africans, people who still live close to the land. Wouldn't you bet their bodies are more congruent than ours?"

"Interesting idea, coming from such a left-brained brain," teases Margie, as she walks back and forth, testing her gait.

"Damn it, Marge," says Bill, his voice rising. He bangs his fist on the coffee table. "You and Kay both. I'm tired of you women acting like you have an option on the right side of the brain."

Fred and Pauline glance at each other. This is a different Bill from the jovial punster they're used to.

Margie stops walking for a moment but otherwise shows no response to Bill's outburst. She takes a few more steps and then an amazed look spreads across her face. She turns and rushes over to Bill, embracing him.

"What the . . . "

"Oh, Bill, thank you," Margie beams. She's breathing hard, as if she'd just run an obstacle course. "You have no idea what you've just done for me."

"Well, kindly clue me in," says poor Bill, embarrassed enough by his outburst and now totally confused by Margie's response.

"It was synchronicity," Margie says. "When you shouted like that, I noticed that I started walking funny on my left foot. Like I was tiptoeing on that side. It all makes sense now."

"You mean because of your parents?" Pauline asks.

"Yes! It must be that whenever I hear angry voices, or maybe whenever I'm under stress, like a lot of pressure at work, I unconsciously try to get everything to quiet down. I'm such a good little helper!"

Margie's eyes are shiny with tears. Bill shuffles his feet and stares at the floor as if looking for a cellar door. Margie reaches out and touches his elbow. "It's okay, Bill. You see, when you showed your feelings, it helped me to find my own. These things might hurt a bit on their way out, but it feels so good to let them go."

"If you say so," Bill says, clearing his throat. "By the way, how come you were humming that tune 'Stand By Me' a while back?"

"Because," Margie answers, sitting down on the sofa, "I'm learning to stand by *me!*"

The group falls silent for a while as they each go inside to sort out their own feelings. A lot has transpired this evening. More than meets the eye, as Bill would say.

"Isn't it amazing?" muses Pauline, breaking the silence. "What a big difference these little changes make when they happen so deep inside your body."

Fred nods. "It's a lot more than just learning to move your body in another way. I thought I knew all there was to know about moving my body. But this gravitational awareness . . ."

"It's 'the path of simplicity.' . . ." Margie settles back.

CHAPTER 9

MY STRUCTURE,
MY SELF

Structural Change as
Energy Transformation

When your structure makes a change toward balance by releasing tension, you experience a transformation of energy. The
transformation can be expressed in many different ways. You may
feel tingling sensations or heat in the area you are focusing on. You
may yawn or sigh or feel a surge of emotion. You may remember
something forgotten, see dreamlike images, or become aware of
sensation elsewhere in your body.

Webster defines energy as the capacity for doing work. Your
body's energy is the work it is accomplishing as it pumps your
blood, fights infection, replaces cells, walks, talks, sweats, and
mows the lawn. A principle of physics called the law of conservation of energy states that while energy may be transformed, it is
never lost. When a baseball player's bat connects with a ball, for
example, mechanical energy of the swing is transformed into
sound and heat. Other forms of energy are light, chemical, atomic,
and electric. All are tools in the body's workshop.

The muscular tension necessary to maintain your body's balance is work—mechanical, chemical, electrical, and atomic energies are spent. To the extent that you do excessive work to support

yourself, you reduce your capacity to spend that energy in other ways. Once you learn to let your structure be supported by gravity, you can stop doing the extra work. The released energy turns first into new sensations, memories, thoughts, or emotions, and then into new ways of working, moving, responding, and being in your body.

When energy has been stored in your body for a long time, its release may be chaotic. Like a dam breaking, your body's localized crisis may reverberate outside local borders. Our planet's ecology is teaching us the global effect of local affairs. Ecological principles hold true within our bodies as well. Lasting structural change both requires and produces changes in every aspect of your being—mental, emotional, and spiritual as well as physical. This is why it's wise to have some strategies for sorting and redirecting the freed energy.

Intrapersonal changes may be facilitated in many ways. The approaches discussed here are Focusing, Process-Oriented Psychotherapy, and Neuro Linguistic Programming. All three use physical sensation to assess change, and their shared tenet—that a release of physical tension accompanies the formation of new attitudes and behavior—fits the well-accepted model of energy conservation.

The discussion of these three approaches to body/mind transformation gives you an introduction to their principles and techniques. These approaches are powerful agents of change. While you may choose to explore any one of these techniques on your own, using this text as a guide, it is most important that you carefully monitor your own experience and seek the guidance of a competent practitioner when necessary

Focusing

Eugene Gendlin's approach to facilitating intrapersonal change developed from many years of investigation of the difference between successful and unsuccessful psychotherapy. Gendlin and his colleagues found that a client's success in therapy had little to do with the technique used but everything to do with the client's physical response to intervention. Patients who experienced psychological change reported an immediate and distinct physical sensation at the moment of insight. Gendlin calls this a "body

MY STRUCTURE,
MY SELF

shift." From his research, this seemed to be the internal requisite that made therapy work.

By studying this physical phenomenon, Gendlin was able to break it down into components he could then teach to clients who didn't naturally check in at the physical level during psychotherapy sessions. Gendlin's practice is to draw a patient's attention to the physical sensations associated with her emotional issue. He calls this physical sensation the "felt sense" of the problem. When the patient acknowledges the physical feeling, and finds words and images to describe it, the felt sense develops and changes in ways that shed light on the original issue.

A distinct change in the felt sense occurs simultaneously with therapeutic insight. The body shift feels like something becoming unstuck or spreading out, like the release you feel after you remember where you left your keys. It's a good feeling, a sense of relief at knowing, even though you may still have to call the locksmith.

Gendlin asserts that your body knows everything it needs to know about being alive in the best possible way. Your body recognizes a feeling of internal "rightness" that enables it to maintain temperature and balance and to repair wounds. Pain or bad feelings indicate potential energy that is pushing toward balance, ease, and comfort.

The six-step Focusing process entails acknowledging an overall, unclear impression of your problem and then letting that impression gradually evolve into a specific quality or image. Once your felt sense has jelled, you may address it with questions as if it were an entity with consciousness. Typical probes might be, "What's the center of this?" or, "What does my felt sense need?"

When your felt sense has changed in response to a question, you then acknowledge the new felt sense and begin another period of questioning. At some point in this process, insight, deep bodily relaxation, and a sense of rightness occur simultaneously. This indicates that your Focusing process is finished.

Focusing might be regarded as an ongoing journey into the interior of your body/mind, with any one felt sense being a visit to a particular place in your internal landscape. Gendlin emphasizes patience, letting the body's internal sense of rightness dictate the pace of change. The interior may be visited again and again, containing, as it does, enough richness and variety of feeling to last a lifetime.

The Focusing technique is the basis for scripts 32 and 34 in the previous chapter. For a detailed self-help manual in this method read Eugene Gendlin's *Focusing*.

Process-Oriented Psychotherapy

Arnold Mindell, the articulator of Process-Oriented Psychotherapy, is a Jungian-based psychotherapist and teacher who became fascinated with the relationship between dreams and bodily phenomena. Mindell discovered that by treating physical symptoms as messages from the unconscious mind, akin to dreams, he was able to aid people in their quest for self-understanding. When symptoms were acknowledged as meaningful rather than merely as conditions to be gotten rid of, they often abated or disappeared. By showing terminally ill patients how to address their illnesses symbolically, Mindell has been able to help these people resolve long-standing life issues and either recover or die peacefully.

Mindell regards the source of the self as a multichanneled entity he calls the "dreambody." The dreambody conveys its information to the conscious mind through the various channels of dreams, physical symptoms and sensations, body language, sounds, visual images, interpersonal relationships, and synchronous events in the world.

One way of understanding a message that comes through your physical channel is to amplify or exaggerate a symptom. Intense focus on the experience of your pain will spontaneously lead to a "channel switch," whereby the pain turns into a sound, movement, or visual image. If insight does not occur at that point, you then amplify the message in the new channel. If your pain turned into a gesture, for example, you could exaggerate the gesture until it either became meaningful or switched to yet another channel. The process is complete when you have gained insight about your problem and are able to express yourself in a new way.

The name Mindell has given to his work—Process-Oriented Psychotherapy, or Process Work—indicates his respect for personal timing and direction. He does not believe that the end of all therapy should be a predetermined ideal of wellness or happiness but that the true quest of any individual is for self-knowledge. Each person's life is a process for which the dreambody provides the map. A therapist's role is to remind the client that the map is available and to offer suggestions for interpreting its symbols. Mindell also believes that resistance should be respected. Resistance to change may signal a premature attempt to force your way into uncharted territory.

By using Mindell's approach in conjunction with the Gravity Game—exaggerating tensions and regarding them as messages, as in script 33—you may address unconscious issues before they turn into symptoms, conceivably nipping potential illness in the bud.

A good reference for learning more about Mindell's approach is his book, *Working with the Dreaming Body*.

Neuro Linguistic Programming

Neuro Linguistic Programming, or NLP, is a description of the structure of human experience rather than psychotherapeutic intervention per se. Its pioneers, John Grinder and Richard Bandler, began by studying qualities that make people successful at human interaction. By observing or modeling people with superior communication skills, they were able to identify specific skills that could then be taught to others. The principles identified by Bandler and Grinder have been expanded by others in many fields. NLP has applications to business, education, politics, and diplomacy as well as to personal change.

One of the basic concepts of NLP is that the contents of your thoughts are less critical to your state of mind than their sequence and the ways they are represented. We represent our experience to ourselves through visual images, sounds, words, and physical impulses. When our way of representing the world becomes habitual, we lose the flexibility to respond freshly to each experience.

Suppose you have a habit of raiding the refrigerator late at night. You've tried everything to stop doing this. You're aware that you're lonely and that you eat to give yourself a feeling of comfort and fullness. Maybe your parents used to bribe you with cookies when they left you with the babysitter. You go into greater and greater detail about why you eat when you're not really hungry, but it makes no difference. You still eat. A feeling of emptiness comes over you that triggers a picture of food, accompanied by stern words reminding you that ice cream is fattening. In no time you're sitting there, spoon in hand.

Through NLP techniques, you can change your relationship to food by altering the way you think about that relationship—the specific sequence of feelings, pictures, and words. After you separate the ways you represent food to yourself, the energy spent keeping them stuck together is freed. This lets you create new responses to your experience. When the lonely feeling no longer automatically triggers a picture of food, it can become a signal for a more productive response. NLP has developed many methods for reprogramming stuck behaviors or beliefs.

Many NLP viewpoints have already been introduced as part of the Gravity Game. One of these is the supposition that a seemingly negative habit comes from a fundamentally positive intention within the person. Most unconscious intentions are in place to protect or to motivate you in some way. If the intention can be accomplished in a different way, the negative behavior may be discarded. Once you learn to feel supported by your legs, you will no longer need to brace your hands on your hips for stability.

Another NLP belief is the importance of a "resource state," or vantage point of comfort and safety from which to view the part of your experience you wish to change. Before processing the food issue mentioned above, for example, one might develop a resource state composed of the sights, sounds, and feelings associated with being emotionally nurtured. Letting your body assume a resourceful state is an important first step in separating yourself from the undesirable and habitual response. It lets you know that things can be different. In the Gravity Game, two resource states that are woven as ongoing themes through all the scripts are fullness of breathing and the feeling of gravitational support.

Another important principle of NLP is "ecology," the idea that any change must respect the integrity of the whole system—body, mind, and spirit. If you change your eating habits but start sniping at your friends, this would indicate that some part of you is not in accord with the change. If a change in the way you use your feet causes pain in your back, then the change is not ecological. Testing for ecology is an integral part of all NLP change methods.

NLP techniques make frequent use of the fact that memory and imagination use the same neurological circuits. Imagination may be used to reframe, or take the sting out of a painful experience, and free your mind for new responses. For such techniques to work, however, the remembered or imagined experiences must be complete with sights, sounds, and feelings. This is called "full representation" of the experience. Your nervous system does not distinguish between reality and imagined experience, if the imagined experience is vivid enough. Ask any kid who has an imaginary friend.

Also built into these techniques is the assumption that the unconscious part of your mind knows what is good for you. If you can learn how to access its advice, it will become a powerful ally.

Three NLP methods that can be helpful in processing structural changes are briefly described below. *Heart of the Mind,* by Connirae and Steve Andreas, and *Frogs into Princes,* by Bandler and Grinder, will give you detailed descriptions of these and other NLP techniques.

Creating Options

Script 33 in chapter 8, in which you were guided to blend the qualities of two sides of your body, was derived from an NLP technique call "the squash." In this practice, you merge two opposing states or behaviors in order to make the dozens of options that lie between them accessible. This amounts to transformation of the energy of the two extremes. Remember that energy cannot be destroyed. The power of the undesirable states can't be discarded, but it can be transformed into more useful or comfortable behaviors.

Suppose one part of you is dedicated to putting others' needs before your own, to seeking harmony and avoiding all conflict. At other times, you find yourself utterly self-absorbed and self-serving. The two parts are like black and white, and you have no control over which part reacts when. The squash technique would give you access to the variety of feelings and behaviors in between those two extremes and the flexibility to respond appropriately to a specific situation.

One way of practicing the squash technique in this situation would be to imagine holding in one hand a full representation of yourself as "doormat"—the sights, sounds, and feelings of yourself in that state. You imagine holding in the other hand a miniature version of your most selfish self. With a steady, relaxed breathing pattern as your resource, you merge the two representations of your self by slowly bringing your two hands together in front of you. You may be aware of some curious neuromuscular twitches in your body as your unconscious mind processes this information. Once your palms have met and your fingers interlace, you bring them to your chest, a ritual that allows the merged representation to settle into your heart.

You can test the result of your squash practice by imagining a situation in which you would ordinarily be inclined to behave one way or the other. If change has penetrated your physiology, the situation will seem to have more options.

Another squash technique is to put vivid representations of each personal quality on two imaginary television screens. Place the TV sets in different parts of the room. You can then walk back and forth between the two qualities/TVs until you feel that the path between them contains new possibilities.

Though these procedures may seem like child's play when you read about them, they are powerful techniques for change. They're effective because they engage both body and mind in re-creating behavior.

Neutralizing
Unpleasant Memories

Sometimes in the course of the Gravity Game processes, an unpleasant memory may surface. An NLP technique that has been dubbed the "phobia cure" is useful for neutralizing painful memories and dislodging their muscular grip on the body.

The first two steps help you dissociate your present time self from the part of you that experienced pain in the past. By establishing distance and safety from your memories, you protect yourself from being overwhelmed by the past sensations.

Begin by imagining yourself in a movie theater. As you sit in your seat you watch yourself on a small black-and-white screen doing some neutral activity like brushing your teeth. Then imagine yourself floating behind your chair so you can watch yourself watching your activities on the screen.

The third step is to watch yourself sitting there watching a black-and-white movie of your unpleasant memory. Watch it from the beginning of the experience all the way to the end, when the unpleasantness is over. When you reach the end, stop the movie so you have a still picture of the experience being over.

The fourth step is to imagine yourself stepping into the still frame, colorizing it, adding dimension and sound, and running it backward very fast. This gives your nervous system the experience of turning time inside out. When you've reached the beginning, think about the memory again. If you can think about it more peacefully, the process is complete. If not, you can repeat the process.

Sometimes a memory of pain persists as an unconscious warning never to let whatever happened occur again. In such a case, just neutralizing the memory would not be ecological. You first need to extract the necessary learning from the memory and integrate it into your present awareness.

One way to extract the learning is through inner dialogue. You might ask yourself, "What do I know now that would have changed my experience if I had known it then?" Or, "What do I know now that would have changed the situation if *they* had known it then?" In either case, go back to the memory and imagine the experience infused with your mature information. If you do this with full representation—sights, sounds, words, movements, and feelings—your nervous system will use this information to detoxify your memory of the experience.

Direction from Your Unconscious Mind

Occasionally feelings surface that are too painful for you to remember consciously. Indications that this is happening would be a feeling of extreme anxiety, sudden inexplicable boredom, or a sense of going blank. This function of your unconscious mind is to protect you from things that would upset your ecology if you knew about them consciously. An NLP technique called "reframing" can help you release tensions that stem from such experiences without necessarily bringing the memory to consciousness.

Reframing describes the process of looking at your experience from a new perspective. In this process, you identify a behavior or tension pattern you wish to change and communicate with it as if it had a personality of its own.

It's easiest to communicate with the part of yourself responsible for your tension if you externalize it—imagine it jumping out in front of your body where you can see and touch it. This aspect of yourself may have recognizable features, but often it will be an abstract shape with seemingly nonsensical qualities. Notice it in detail—its texture, shape, color, temperature, and weight. Notice whether there is a sound associated with your externalized part. Does it have a voice? Is the voice high-, medium-, or low-pitched? Does it sound familiar? Ask this aspect of yourself in charge of the tension to let you know what its intention for you is.

When you have received its message, give your heartfelt thanks. Then explain that while you appreciate its hard work, you'd like to have more freedom in your body. Ask the part in charge if it would be okay to accomplish the intention in a different way. Most tensions will be happy to be relieved of the responsibility of doing the same thing all the time and will agree to the prospect of finding new alternatives.

Then ask the creative part of yourself to concoct dozens of other ways of satisfying the intention. It will do this in your unconscious mind too fast for you to keep track of every choice. Ask it to let you know when it's finished creating alternatives.

When the choices have been created, ask the aspect in charge of the tension to go shopping for new alternatives. You'll feel a response in your body when it has selected some good ones. You may or may not consciously know what they are.

Return your attention to the aspect of yourself you've been holding in your hands. Notice any changes in its characteristics— shape, color, temperature, tone of voice. Thank it for being willing to try some new ways of carrying out its purpose. Then take it back into yourself by bringing your hands to your chest or by inhaling it back inside.

The last step in this process is to scan your whole body/mind system for ecology. Is there any other part of you that objects to this change? Is there tension somewhere else in your body? If so, you can then establish communication with the objecting part and repeat the reframing process with it.

Features of Body/Mind Processing

Before picking up this book, you may have already embarked along a satisfying psychological or spiritual path. You may be looking for a new approach or a different therapist. Or you may have started out just wanting help for your body and are surprised to find yourself involved in affairs of the mind and heart. Whatever your stage of personal evolution, you may occasionally need professional assistance.

Gendlin's and Mindell's work and NLP each embody three important beliefs or features that make for effective body/mind therapy or self-help processes. These common threads can be used as guidelines when you interview a prospective therapist. Consider the following questions when you look for help.

Does the therapist's approach acknowledge the inherent wisdom of your unconscious body/mind? All three of the approaches described above answer yes to this question.

Does the movement toward change honor the ecology of the whole body/mind/spirit system? Mindell's process-oriented approach and Gendlin's patience with small shifts of the felt sense are examples of ecological orientation. The safety provided by the NLP concept of a resource state is another aspect of ecology. It insures that the small, painful part of yourself under examination is not mistaken for the whole.

All three approaches also acknowledge resistance to change and provide the opportunity for possible unconscious resistance to be expressed. The last step of the NLP reframing process has you check your whole body/mind system for any objection to the changes you have made. Change is not ecological until the objecting part has been integrated.

Does the approach respect the law of conservation of energy? All three of the methods described follow a pattern of sorting experience through various channels or representational systems. When the visual images, sounds, feelings, and movements that have been stuck together around an experience can be sorted and separated, there follows a release of energy that allows insight and new behavior to occur. No symptom, feeling, bad habit, or tension can simply be discarded, but when its positive intention or message is integrated, change occurs spontaneously.

A fourth principle of effective body/mind therapy has become evident through structural integration methods like Rolfing and Rolfing Movement. This involves establishing physical support for nonphysical change. The sensation of gravitational support for the body translates to the mind as stability and security. Thus, gravity is an invaluable safety net for the sometimes scary moments when you're letting go of the muscular bracing from a painful experience.

Sometimes releasing an old habit feels as if the rug has been pulled out from under you or as if boundaries have disappeared. If a new pattern of bracing develops, it indicates that ecological principles are being violated. But if the balanced support of gravity is established as a resource, you then have a comfortable physical home in which to lodge your new attitudes and behaviors.

The Gravity Gang

"Bill's having a hard time, isn't he?" Pauline asks. She and Margie are taking a walk. It's several days after their get-together with Bill and Fred.

"Yes and no," Margie replies. "He's made a lot of headway since Kay left him—that jolt really made him take a look at himself. But 'headway' is what it mostly is so far. He only seems to want to change his appearance, and he thinks he can do it by reading a book."

"I think he's more aware of his feelings than you give him credit for, Margie. And I also think he gets under your skin somehow."

"You're right about that. Funny how he kept inadvertently helping me the other night. I couldn't remember the name of that song for anything, and he tuned right in to my own unconscious pun." Margie has her arms crossed now and is taking bold strides, landing hard on her heels. Pauline has to hurry to keep up. Suddenly Margie stops. "There I am with this big insight about standing up for myself, feeling my own center, reclaiming my space, and right in the middle of telling him how great it all is I notice the old holding-back pattern in my chest. I stood there bracing myself just like I am right now!"

"Like this?" Pauline asks, copying Margie's stance. "Give yourself a break, Margie. And give Bill one too. This stuff takes time. You're literally peeling off layers of defense, and you can't be expected to have it all together. You act like you think you should have achieved nirvana yesterday."

Margie lets out a big sigh and drops her arms. "You're a wise young woman, Paulie," she says. "Thanks for the reminder. I guess I could get as obsessive about gravity as anything else—job, clothes, money, men, fitness—I've tried them all. Maybe this time I'll get the message."

"What do you think the message is?" Pauline asks.

"Well, I think part of it is that being supported by gravity gives you an internal compass. It's a way of knowing where you are inside. Once you know what centeredness feels like, you can tell when you're off."

"An automatic congruency gauge."

"That's it. The heaviness or lightness of your body keeps you in touch with your feelings."

"I like your compass idea," Pauline says, "just as long as you don't use it to jerk yourself around."

"Not much danger with you around," Margie replies. "Now what about you? You didn't just have an attack of the munchies the other night. What happened?"

"Well, Bill was reading the script about merging the two sides of the body, and I got this big red stop sign. I didn't so much see it as feel it—a sinking sensation in the pit of my stomach. It was like a big, bottomless hole."

Pauline's pace has slowed down as she talks, and Margie watches her friend's face lose its color. "Sounds like it wasn't something you'd want to leap into."

"Not then, anyway. But I would like to explore it," Pauline says. "Wow. We're on our street already. I lost track of where we were." She blinks her eyes a few times and tosses her head. "Guess I lost my compass for a minute."

"You know," Margie reflects after a pause, "when you think about it, each one of us is just a piece of the earth. It's like we're squatters in our own little tracts of land. Strange how easy it is to get lost."

"Margie, have you read that section about the NLP reframing process?"

"Yes," Margie says as the two climb the steps to their apartment. "Seems like that might help you sort this out. Would you like some help on Saturday?"

"It's a date," Pauline smiles, fitting her key into the lock.

It's Saturday morning. Margie tosses a log on the fire while Pauline stretches out on a rug in front of the fireplace. "What a cozy way to spend a rainy morning," Pauline muses.

Settling herself on a cushion beside her roommate, Margie watches the fire while Pauline tunes into her breathing.

"How's your body feeling?" Margie asks after a few minutes.

"Good. I feel my dimensions, and I feel supported. My right leg seems a tiny bit heavier than my left, but it isn't a big deal. What I notice most is that my breathing takes a detour around my lower abdomen. Kind of like a river going around a boulder in midstream."

"Have you ever noticed that before?"

"Sure. It's the same place that I'm forever longing to get rid of. Sit-ups don't seem to help."

"Well, let that place know that you're not trying to get rid of it anymore, that you'd like to get acquainted and maybe even help it do whatever it's doing for you."

Pauline's face takes on a faraway look as she hears these words. After a moment her belly gurgles loudly and she laughs. "We just had breakfast. I can't be hungry."

"Maybe your stomach is saying something."

Pauline is silent. She hears another gurgle or two. At last she sighs and nods. "The boulder is softer now, almost as if it liked being acknowledged."

"Then let's see if we can communicate with it. If you could take the boulder outside your body and hold it in your hands in front of you, what would its characteristics be?"

Pauline is quiet for a long time. The muscles of her brow and lower jaw fluctuate slightly, letting Margie know that her friend is watching internal pictures. "That was amazing," Pauline says at last. "For a while I just saw a bunch of shapes and flashes of light. Then for a second I saw our Christmas dinner table with all my relatives sitting around, me—real little—my cousins, and my uncle, the one who used to tease me. . . ."

She pauses again and her brow darkens. Then with a sigh she continues. "Then everything went blank and there was just this big box, all wrapped up like a present."

"Well," says Margie, "ask the present if it will communicate with you."

"Yes," says Pauline, without hesitation.

"How do you know that?"

"Because the wrapping paper started to sparkle and the bow sort of lit up."

"Can you make it do that on purpose?"

"Yes," Pauline says after a few moments. "But it isn't the same."

"Ask your present if it will tell you what's inside," suggests Margie.

"It's just a big, silly package now," Pauline says. "It won't budge."

"Well, that's a kind of communication, isn't it?"

Pauline chuckles. "I thanked it and it said, 'You're welcome.' I guess it's not ready to reveal any secrets."

"Ask the present if it would be willing to find some other ways of doing whatever it's doing for you, so you wouldn't have to keep that tension in your tummy all the time."

Pauline nods.

"Okay, Pauline," Margie says softly. "You know the next two steps. Ask the present to explain its purpose to the creative part of your unconscious mind. Then ask your creativity to dream up lots and lots of other ways of achieving that purpose, so many ways that you can't consciously keep track of them. Let me know when you're finished with the process."

Pauline is quiet for several minutes. Her face, though rosy, is almost without expression save for a faint smile. Margie is beginning to wonder if her friend's attention has wandered. Then Pauline swallows. "That was something," she says dreamily. "There was this Christmas tree with colored lights—that was my creative part making up alternatives. I knew it was finished when the lights stopped blinking."

"Good. Now ask the package to choose at least three new responses it can use the next time its intention is necessary. Let it signal you when it's done choosing."

In just a few moments Pauline nods.

"Now scan your whole body and see if there's any part of you that objects to the new choices."

Pauline seems to be holding her breath, and her face looks strained. Then she sighs. "I felt a pressure on my thighs," she says. "It was like a shadow. But I kept breathing and it got lighter, and then it sort of drifted off behind me. I can still see it way back there."

"Does it have an objection?"

"No. But it wants to stay there in the background," says Pauline. "The tension in my belly is gone though."

"Maybe you should do a few pelvic rolls," suggests Margie, "to let your body get used to moving without that old tension."

Pauline's interest in pelvic rolls is half-hearted. She's eager to get up and move around with the new feeling. She rolls over and stands up. "Whoa," she exclaims, "that feels too strange!" The color has suddenly drained from her face.

Margie pulls up a chair and gestures for Pauline to sit. "We'd better do some integration. I think you were engaging in some important personal work, even though it seemed like a Christmas party."

"Yes, I feel like my legs have disappeared. That advice about integrating the changes physically—that must be more important than I thought." Pauline concentrates, rocking her body forward and back, exploring her sitting zone. "Now I feel my weight settling into my pelvis. There's more room in there than before."

"Lean forward just a little so the weight of your legs can rest into your feet."

"Yes, that's better," Pauline says.

Margie, watching, has the impression that Pauline is taking up new residence in the lower half of her body. "That feels grounded, more stable now," Pauline says.

"I've never seen you look so comfortable sitting down, Pauline."

"It's true. Usually I'm curling my legs underneath me and squirming all over the place."

"Try standing up. Rock forward into your feet and push up to standing. Keep that open feeling in your pelvis. . . . Wow. Did that feel as easy as it looked?"

The women are interrupted by the doorbell. "I'll get that," Margie says, starting toward the hall. "Why don't you try a few knee bends?"

I remember feeling I was at home in my body a few weeks ago, Pauline thinks to herself, but that was nothing compared to this. She bends her knees, feeling her weight settle into her feet with complete trust. The degree of trust feels new. Her breath moves smoothly through her pelvis. It seems to her as though maybe something bad might have happened when she was very small. But she has an odd feeling of protection now, as if she needn't remember it until she's ready. As her feet press into the carpet, she feels her body rise without effort, calm and sure and centered. She walks over to give Fred a hug.

"Say," says Fred, "something nice has been going on here. I can feel it down inside your skin."

"Like I'm softer?" asks Pauline.

"Hold on, you two," interrupts Margie. "Let's make sure Pauline feels finished before we wrap this up."

"I feel great," says Pauline. "I feel *present*. Present in my legs and pelvis in a brand new way. Do you think maybe we withdraw our spirit from parts of the body where we've experienced some kind of trouble?"

"What do you think?"

"Well, before my legs and belly were tense all the time and I didn't even know it. Like I was both uptight and not there. Numb, I guess. Maybe the tension was a way to make boundaries for myself. So when I stood up too fast a moment ago, it felt like the boundaries were gone along with the tension."

"That was scary."

"Yes. But then I got back in touch with gravity—at a deeper level of awareness than before. Support feels more supporting and dimension feels fuller, so I can just sort of settle down inside myself and relax."

"You know," muses Margie, "the earth has been here all along. And she's not going to let go of us for a while."

"You mean we might as well accept her help and stop straining so hard to hold ourselves up?"

"Sort of reframes the game, doesn't it?" Margie answers, nodding. "Give me a hug too, will you?"

"Thanks, Margie. That was more help than you know."

"Can I say 'Hi' now?" asks Fred when the two women turn his way.

"Sorry for ignoring you," Margie says. "How've you been?"

"Well, I think I'm becoming a gravity convert at last. That exercise the other night changed some things for me."

"Like what?"

"Oh, after paying so much attention to my knee the other night, I've started noticing how much tension I store in my right leg. It turns out I've been gripping my thighs and butt when I'm driving. Since I spend so much time on the road, that's a lot of gripping. So guess what?"

The women look at him expectantly.

"I realized that you don't really need to work your whole leg to press down on the gas pedal. Just flex your ankle—such a simple solution. Then I moved the seat-back forward and that made it easier to release the weight of my torso into my pelvic basin. When I let go of the unnecessary tension in my hips, presto, no more back pain!"

"Three cheers for gravity," says Margie, beaming.

"That's great!" says Pauline, moving close for another hug. "Your insides feel different too!"

"I have an idea," says Margie, when the excitement dies down. "We've been talking so much about how good it feels to occupy our bodies in this new way. How about practicing what we preach while we preach it? I mean we could practice our gravity awareness while we're talking to each other. What do you say?"

"What'll we talk about?" asks Fred, looking unenthusiastic.

"Doesn't matter. Anything."

"I have a better idea," says Pauline. "I'll sing for you."

Fred and Margie struggle to keep from looking dumbfounded. Pauline has always been very private about her singing, always refusing their requests with a modest "I'm not ready." Something's changed and they're delighted. Their pleasure soars as they listen to their friend sing—first a few operatic arias and then some Gershwin songs. Her voice seems to resonate from the soles of her feet.

"Well, that's it," Pauline smiles, ejecting her accompaniment tape from the cassette player. Raindrops spatter against the windows.

"Pauline, your voice is beautiful," Margie beams. "You can't just hide it away. It's a gift!"

Bill has set aside the evening to play the tape Margie made when he read the scripts to the others on Sunday night. She always thinks of everything, just like his mother packing him off to school. Well, now he has no excuse to put off the nitty gritty. Fred and Margie seemed to have gotten a lot out of it, though Margie's enthusiasm can be exhausting at times. But no question that Fred looked less lopsided at the end of the evening—that was impressive.

Bill switches on his desk lamp and sets his tape recorder down. He's glad to be working by himself, especially after lashing out at Marge and making her cry. He can't imagine what got into him. Sometimes he just can't get a handle on his feelings, can't find the right words. Sometimes words come so easily, and other times the wrong ones come tumbling out. He had the same trouble with Kay. He sighs and picks up a pile of books and magazines lying on the floor beside the couch. He idly flips pages of a computer journal, then glances at his worn copy of Robert Frost. "The way out is through," he mutters. "You said that somewhere, didn't you, old man?"

Stretching out on the carpet, Bill gradually relaxes. Aware of the silence in the house, he thinks fleetingly of Kay and wonders how she's spending the evening. Sternly he jerks his attention back to business at hand. He turns on the tape and starts breathing. After a while it seems to him as though something is pushing down on his shoulders. It's tight around his chest too, and he can't get a full breath. Weeks ago, he remembers, a similar thing had happened, right here in his den. "Okay," he mutters, "*through.*"

Bill sits up to get a better sense of what his body is trying to tell him. It's as if someone, or something, is pushing down on his shoulders, and there's a heavy feeling across his back. He puts his own hands on his shoulders and pushes down, attempting to intensify the sensation.

"We all have our cross to bear," he hears. It's his father's voice, harsh and distant. And Bill is curled up, hiding in a small, dark place. Bill's eyes are closed now, and he lets himself curl up into the posture of his younger self long ago. Where is he?

"Oh," Bill sighs. "I remember." He stretches out again on the rug and lets the memory flood past. He'd grown up in a religious family, and his father was especially strict. As an altar boy, Bill used to get up before dawn and bicycle alone to church to prepare for early mass. The church would be populated with strange shadowy shapes. He'd hurry to the altar where he felt safe near the statue of the Holy Mother. One morning he'd nodded off staring at her face and was startled by the sound of heavy footsteps. Half asleep, he'd been terrified and dived under the altar draperies where he hid for the rest of the morning until all the services were done. When he finally got home, his father had spanked him mercilessly for playing hooky.

It was all a big mistake. He'd been afraid, and then embarrassed at his fear, scared to let the priest know that he was hiding under the sacred altar and mortified at having his father find out. His secret sin grew heavier and heavier, like a big cross. And he'd carried that burden long after he'd forgotten about it, long after he'd left organized religion and embraced a more private relationship with his God. And the burden was still with him every time he did something embarrassing.

Bill takes as big a breath as he can and blows it out through

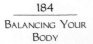

his lips, letting the crazy sound it makes interrupt his reverie. "Steady now," he says to himself. "You can just stand next to this old memory and look inside. It won't bite."

Breathing now, Bill still feels some restriction across his chest and shoulders and back. It's heavy, like armor. Bill tries to appreciate his tension, to believe in some positive purpose for feeling the way he does. But it's difficult. He hates the restricted feeling and he wants out.

Returning to his childhood memory, Bill asks himself what he knows now that would have helped him if he'd known it back then. How could he have responded differently to the situation?

Looking for a key to unlock his rusty armor, Bill runs a movie of the childhood scene—the dark church, the dive under the altar, hiding, his father's anger—all the way to the end when the spanking is forgotten and he's okay again. He watches the movie a second time, in black and white and faster so everything looks jerky, like an old silent film. And then he plays it backward, putting himself inside the film and zipping backward through time. Whoooosh. He does it again and again. Now it's becoming funny to watch himself materialize feet first from beneath the altar. He could almost laugh. Well, at least he's not holding his breath any more, and he can look back at the experience more objectively.

It occurs to Bill now that he could have come out of hiding as soon as he realized the footsteps belonged to Father Paisley. The priest would have understood he was just a sleepy little boy. And suppose he hadn't. Bill laughs out loud as he pictures himself lecturing the priest about compassion. What's funny is that the little boy has grown-up Bill's deep voice.

Bill gets up and shuffles down the hall for some milk and crackers. He sits at the kitchen table staring into space. Dreamily, he watches a little boy pulling a red wagon. Inside the wagon is a big, heavy cross. The little boy pulls the wagon way back into the past, back to where Bill's father is standing. "Dad," the boy says, "I believe this cross belongs to you. I found it, and I don't need it anymore." The boy shakes his father's hand, turns, then sails into the kitchen and bites down on a cracker.

"Wow," says Bill, squirming and straightening up. "Got to do something about these chairs. They make your buns go to sleep." He stands up and absentmindedly slaps his buttocks. "Holy smokes!"

Now Bill strides excitedly back and forth across the room, stopping every so often to bend his knees and wag his hips. "Sitting bones, you're free now. No more spankings for you."

Getting ready for bed, Bill glances at himself in the mirror. There's new breadth across his chest, and he looks longer from his hips to his shoulders. He's going to have to start watching out for doorways now that he's riding so tall. He bends his knees again. Sure enough! His body weight settles down into his pelvis just like sitting on a saddle. He remembers the shape of the pelvic bones. "So my buttocks don't have to grip at all. If I keep this up, I'll have to buy new jeans."

Standing there in his boxers, Bill takes a deep, free breath. For the first time in years, he feels like dancing.

CHAPTER 10

WINNING THE GAME

"You're looking great, Bill," Fred says, clapping the other man on the shoulder. "Haven't seen you for a long time. When was that?"

"About six months ago, I guess. You don't look so bad yourself."

"Thanks. I feel good. Glad we're getting together, though. I can use the review."

"It can't hurt. This gravity stuff has done a lot for me. Did Pauline tell you Kay and I have gotten back together?"

"Yes. She said you're taking dancing lessons or something." Fred makes his way to the couch.

"Greek dancing—it's great. Kay always wanted me to go folk dancing with her, but I felt too clumsy. But now I feel like," Bill clicks his heels together and snaps his fingers, "a new man."

Fred chuckles. "So gravity turned you into a Greek, huh?"

"Better Greek than geek!" Bill mimes a double take and looks around menacingly. "Who said that?"

Fred shrugs his shoulders. "Your alter ego maybe?"

"Well, show him the door." Bill joins Fred on the sofa. "Say, Margie tells me you and Pauline are pretty tight these days."

"I guess you could say that. We're both very busy right now. She's got a new job, and I'm still on the road a lot. But when we do have time together, it's magic."

"Speaking of magic," Bill says, "that pelvic-roll motion has done great things for Kay and me—for our sex life, I mean."

"We noticed that too," Fred smiles. "There seems to be no end to the benefits of the Gravity Game."

"I may just owe my marriage to gravity," Bill remarks. The two men lean back, smiling. Bill seems about to confide something more when Margie walks in.

"Hi, guys."

"Hi, Margie."

"Great idea to get us together to review those gravity moves, Marge," Bill says, winking at Fred.

"How come?" Margie asks, sensing she's missed a beat.

"Well, . . . because I've been having a headache lately. For the past week I've had this nagging pain at the nape of my neck."

"What's going on?" Margie asks. "You've had headaches before, haven't you?"

"Yes. I used to get them a lot before I raised the height of my screen at work. Computers wreak havoc on people's bodies, you know that."

"But your workstation fits your body now, so that can't be it. Have you been doing anything differently in the last week?"

"Not really. Just a new exercise video—I've been doing more push-ups." Bill puffs out his pecs. Because of his old habit of slouching, Bill's upper chest has never been very well developed. Now that he feels better about himself, he's more comfortable with that part of his body and eager to develop it further.

"That just might be the problem, though," offers Fred. "Show us how you do those push-ups."

Bill gets down on the floor to demonstrate.

"Bill, it looks like you're only using the muscles in your arms and upper shoulders to push with," suggests Fred. "Stop for a second. Get in touch with your shoulder blades, feel how they connect your arms to your back. Now, push up using the undersides of your arms."

"That's a lot harder," Bill complains. "It makes my back do more of the work, and I can't do as many."

"Not until your back and shoulders get stronger. But notice how much broader your chest is."

"You're right," Bill says.

"If you work with your chest broad, then you'll develop a broad chest. But if you work narrow, you'll just reinforce your old pattern," explains Fred.

"You know what else? My neck feels more at ease when I do it this way. I think I've been clenching my neck and jaw to do these push-ups."

"So maybe that's the source of your headache."

"Another round for gravity," quips Margie.

"Thanks a lot, you two." Bill stands up and tucks in his shirt.

"Glad to help," says Fred. "But listen, let's not do any more work until Pauline gets here. She'd hate to miss anything."

"Okay by me." Bill turns to Fred. "Say, Fred, what's with the van? I thought you and that red Corvette were like a married couple."

"Well, no matter how I tinkered with the seat, I never could get it to fit just right. The van is a lot more comfortable. Besides, I need the room for some kids I know."

"Say, Margie told me you've been doing some kind of volunteer work. What's that all about?"

"I've been teaching some bodybuilding classes at a center for disabled kids. You know, those little guys can enjoy their bodies too, even though they don't operate like everybody else's."

"How did you get into that?"

"Well, it may sound strange, but the last time we got together—remember that script about getting messages from your body?—I won't go into the whole story, but I saw this big sign that said 'Boys' Club.' One thing led to another, and I ran into this place."

"Far out," says Bill. "Did you ever think of doing anything like that before?"

"No. I was always too busy trying to prove myself at one thing or another. But that night, I saw how I'd been compensating for some mean things I did to my brother when we were kids. So this project is a way of balancing it out—making amends if you will."

"It must be satisfying."

"More than anything I've ever done."

"You know," Bill says, "a year ago I never would have believed that you could make changes in your life just by tuning in to your body."

The Trophy Is Your Body

Your game with gravity should develop into an ongoing and self-perpetuating attitude of play. It is not a contest you try to win, with a trophy to display on a shelf. If there is a trophy, it's your body, and as long as you're alive and kicking, the trophy keeps changing in its process of dynamic relationship with the earth. Hopefully this book has made you aware of this dynamic relationship and has given you some tips about making it as graceful, responsive, and comfortable a relationship as possible.

The principles you're now acquainted with are powerful. They'll rehabilitate and maintain your physical structure throughout your days, so that when you've grown old and experienced enough to have become wise, you'll still be agile and strong enough to share your wisdom.

What have you learned? To breathe—to sense the movement of your breath connecting every part of your body with every other part. The flow of your breath signals to you where you have created a barrier in your body, where stress or incongruency have invaded your system. Your breath also gives your body the stability of three dimensions. You operate in wholeness, not as parts or sides.

You've also learned what support feels like. You have sentient understanding of the earth beneath your feet. No praise or possession can compare with the personal security of knowing where you stand. And you know your center, the core of your physical self. You know the difference between feeling tight to the bone, braced against life's experiences, and having a core that responds freely to the experience of the present moment. You know the feeling of support in your pelvis as well as in your feet. And the feeling of having plenty of room in your pelvis for your fundamental instincts, for your gut feelings. You have a sense of the fluency of your joints, of their democratic sharing of responsibility for your motion. You've learned to recognize a sense of integration when you initiate the movements of your limbs from your spine. Arms, legs, and head radiate from your core like the points of a starfish from its center. You know when your head, heart, and gut are congruent.

When It's Time
for a Tune-Up

The kids are sick, you've missed a deadline, your car has been burglarized, your favorite team lost a big game, and your mother-in-law is visiting for a month. Let gravity help you sort things out. Close the door for ten minutes and listen to one or two of the following scripts:

> Script 5—Exploring Your Back Half
> Script 16—Integrative Knee Bends
> Script 21—Pelvic Roll, Roll to Standing,
>   Knee Bends
> Script 22—Activating Your Suspender Muscles
> Script 23—Moving from Sitting to Standing
> Script 32—Movement Mantra

Though any of the Gravity Game scripts can be useful for maintaining your structural awareness, these several are especially recommended. You may be surprised at the centering effect of these movement meditations. By focusing your attention inside your structure, you re-attune yourself to your personal path of simplicity. Focused attention lets you separate the wheat from the chaff. Maybe you'll miss breakfast during that ten-minute break, but you'll suddenly remember that today is your spouse's birthday. It's not too late to make reservations at a favorite restaurant, and Mom can take care of the kids.

As you review any pattern, remind yourself that its goal is the sensation of ease and support. The difference in sensation *may* create a different shape in the mirror, but don't measure your success on visual feedback. Let sensation guide your changes.

The sensations of your balanced relationship with gravity are your biggest assets in this ongoing game. Sometimes, when you can't take time out for a tune-up, just remembering the important sensations will be enough to relieve your stress, recover your center, and set you moving on a balanced track again.

Remember to cultivate a friendly attitude toward your old habits. Appreciate them for the support they've given you in the past. Seduce them into helping you by putting them in charge of developing new ways to cope with your stresses. Listen to their messages.

Perhaps at some point you'll receive a message you would rather not have heard or recognize some painful aspect of yourself or your history that you'd just as soon ignore. Remember that *you* are not your pain. With the support engendered by your new relationship with gravity, you can move to one side of your pain. Breathing calmly, let the earth support you as you observe that pain in a new light and reframe its meaning.

Set time aside to choreograph some of your daily routines—the way you perform your tasks, the simple motions of reaching, bending, looking, turning, and walking. Notice where gravity supports your intentions and where you sabotage your ease with counterintentions in your body. Pick one specific action to redesign. Then practice one or two of the Gravity Game patterns to remind yourself of the feeling of ease and support. Afterward, ask yourself the question, "How can I perform *this* task with *that* feeling in my body?"

Visualization is another way to redesign your daily activities. First, practice a couple of the Gravity Game patterns to heighten your structural awareness. Then visualize yourself in your work situation, on the golf course, on the dance floor, in the weight room, in the swimming pool—in whatever activity you'd like to change relative to the way you use your body. Picture the scene in living color, with textures, temperatures, and sound. Research has shown that thought produces measurable electrochemical changes in the body. Your mental rehearsal of a different way of behaving actually creates new behavior.

It's most important that you give yourself time to learn these new ways of being in your body. Appreciate the power of small changes. A tiny change truly integrated into your daily responses will gather momentum. Coax your structure into centeredness during those few moments when you're brushing your teeth. That simple morning reminder will come back to you in the cafeteria line and will help transform the way you stand your ground anywhere.

Yet another way of improving your structure is to tune in to your own best relationship to gravity. Remember a time when you were in a very self-confident state, when you felt grounded, flexible, spontaneous, and secure. It might be some recent time or a moment long ago. Once you have a clear memory of that time, re-create that physical state. Let your body feel it again in the present. Then begin moving about, savoring the ease and stability.

Notice your support, dimension, core, fluidity, and congruency as you walk, bend, sit, and stand.

You can also improve your structure by assuming the physical state of someone else who moves comfortably and gracefully: a child, a dancer, an athlete. Let your body model their moves, but concentrate on the *feeling* rather than the look of the movement.

The Gravity Game should make life easier, not weigh you down with details. So if you're one of those people for whom six things to remember—breathing, support, dimension, core, fluidity, and congruency—is five too many, pick number one: breathing. Just breathe. Let your elbows breathe, your knees, your eyes, your baby toes. And maybe you'll remember just one other comment or idea from this book that spoke to your body, that seemed to make a difference. Six months from now, when your body is different, you might run across this book again. Perhaps another idea will ring true then. There is no rush. You have a lifetime to get comfortable inside your skin.

The Gravity Gang

"Hi, everybody. I've got incredible news!" Pauline appears at the door with her arms outspread as if making a stage entrance. Her hair is piled high on top of her head, and she's wearing a colorful, gypsylike outfit.

Bill whistles. "Here's a sight for sore eyes. I didn't know you were in a play, Pauline."

"Hi, Bill. Gosh, it's gravity night, isn't it? Oh, Margie, Fred! I'm so excited. Guess who came in tonight?" Pauline sails around the room hugging everyone. Then she stands back in a vain attempt at composure. Her news tumbles out all in one breath. "These producers, they're doing a revival of *Kiss Me Kate* at the Grand and they liked my singing and they want me to try out for the part of Kate!" She picks up her long skirts and twirls. "I'm so excited!"

"That's fantastic, Paulie," beams Fred. "What a break!"

"And Lucky was so proud that he got Carla to clear my station and let me come home early. So here I am. Oh . . ."

"Will somebody please fill me in," says Bill. "Who's Lucky?"

"Lucky's the owner of Luciano's," explains Margie. "That's where Pauline works. It's a cabaret. When he found out she could sing, he made her part of the show, so she serves dinner and then she sings. Lots of singers have gotten started there."

"I'm going to get out of these clothes," Pauline says. "Be back in a minute. Sorry I kept you guys waiting."

"Worth every minute," says Fred.

"No problem," calls Bill. "I didn't even know she could sing," he says, turning to the others. "She has made some changes!"

"We all have," Margie says. "That's why I wanted to get us all together again."

"Well, how are we going to do this?" asks Bill.

"I thought we'd just share with one another the discoveries we've made and any quandaries we might have and then maybe review some of the gravity patterns."

"Sounds like a good plan," says Bill.

For the next few minutes, Margie, Fred, and Bill help themselves to snacks and get comfortable. Pauline rejoins them, wearing jeans and scrubbed of her glamorous makeup but still radiant.

"I'll start the ball rolling," offers Bill. "The big thing for me is taking gravity breaks. I used to meditate, you know. I still do sometimes, but this is different. When I do a tune-up, it seems to bring my body and mind into synch in a way that feels . . . gosh, how to explain it?"

"When I do them, I feel more present," comments Fred.

"Right. Meditation makes me feel detached from my stress. But this gets me feeling detached and present in my body at the same time. It's great. I find solutions to problems, get new ideas and inspiration, not to mention relaxation and this handsome new body . . ."

"Sounds like we could start a cult if we're not careful," warns Fred.

"What's great about it," Margie breaks in, "is that you can use this practice for all different levels of working on yourself. Sometimes it seems to foster just a physical change. Other times you find an emotional pattern in your body, and that gives you a chance to know yourself better. And still other times, you get in touch with a peaceful center—I suppose that's finding your spiritual self."

"Gravity's gifts to us," muses Pauline, staring at the fire. Then she looks at the others. "I've got something to share. Now that I'm singing popular music, I have to use my arms more expressively than I did for concert performing. At first I felt like such a ham, and my arms felt like props that had nothing to do with me. But gradually I'm learning how to let my gestures come from the same source as my voice. It all wells up from the earth, up through my body and out my heart."

"That's beautiful," says Fred, giving her an admiring smile.

"It is when I find it," says Pauline. "And I'm starting to map out the way to get there. It feels just like walking does when everything's congruent. There's no difference between my upper body and my lower body. Relaxing my arms makes my legs feel more alive and visa versa."

"I get that feeling once in a while on the tennis court," Bill remarks. "It's great. Hey, you'll give us a song in a little while, won't you?"

"Sure, Bill, a special one just for you," smiles Pauline.

"Well, gang," says Fred, "let me show you something I'm struggling with." He stands up and moves in front of the fireplace. "I've still got that imbalance in my hips. It's better than it was, but lately I've noticed that I spend a lot more time standing on my right leg than my left. Remember that evaluation in the beginning of the book, when you stand as if you were waiting in line? Well, look, and tell me what you see." Fred rests his weight first on his right side, then on his left.

"When you're standing on the left, you look kind of uncertain," comments Bill. "Not as if you're going to fall over or anything, but . . ."

"But compared to the right—" says Margie, "when you're on the right, you look like you're at home."

"And that's how it feels," says Fred. "So what do I do about it?"

"What do you do when you find yourself standing on your dominant leg?" asks Margie.

"Usually I correct myself and stand evenly on both feet."

"Right. So you're acting like a stern parent." Margie knits her brows and shakes a finger at Fred. "Now, how many times have I told you not to stand on that leg?" she says in a grating tone. "But that strategy doesn't really work, does it?"

"I guess not."

"I bet you're not acknowledging your strong leg for the good job it's been doing. Instead you're scolding it for being so strong. And when you try to impose a different attitude on your body, naturally your body rebels."

"Margie, remember that blending process we explored?" Pauline breaks in. "Do you think that might help Fred with this imbalance?"

"You mean when you blended your different sitting options?" Pauline nods.

"Sure. Give it a try."

"Okay, I told you about this, remember Freddie? I was having trouble finding a comfortable way to sit at the piano. What I did was move very, very slowly back and forth between my usual arched-forward position and a wider, more open feeling in my pelvis."

"I remember. So I need to blend my stance, right?" Fred leans on his right side, knee locked, arms folded across his chest. His left foot rests lightly on the floor.

"Okay," Pauline says. "Now, very, very slowly, start rising up out of your right hip and shift some of your weight over into the left side of your pelvis. . . . That's it. You might have to draw your left foot in a little closer. Keep going, but slow down even more. It helps you feel it if you close your eyes. . . . Let some weight go down your left leg into your foot. Keep going until you feel like you're standing evenly on both. And remember to breathe. . . ."

"How's this?"

"How does it feel?" Pauline responds.

"A little strange—not bad though." A wrinkle plays across Fred's forehead as he focuses on the unfamiliar sensations.

"Great. Now, just as slowly, go back where you started from. And remember, it's okay to breathe. . . . That's it—just let your weight gradually drift over onto your right side again. Let yourself feel the tiny gradations of change all along the way."

When Fred has returned to his original stance, Pauline asks him to repeat the process. The second time around he spontaneously drops his arms but keeps his hands clasped loosely together. With his eyes closed, it's as if he can see each side of his body from within. It's odd how different they seem—the right feels dense and strong, but resistant too, as if it were the home for his stubborn streak. By contrast, his whole left side seems airy, like he hasn't spent much time living over there. He continues swaying, noticing the border between his two internal territories. There's a kind of buzzing deep inside his body each time he crosses that border and once he jerks involuntarily.

Fred continues his exploration, an absorbed look on his face.

The others wait, knowing he's learning something important about himself from the sensations inside his body.

When Fred finally stops, his weight balanced between his two sides, he releases his hands and takes a deep breath. "This feels good," he says, opening his eyes.

"What did you find out?" Pauline asks.

"Well, at first I thought there were only two possible 'homes,'" Fred answers, "my habitual stance and a better, more balanced one. But by moving that slowly, I could feel what a stranger I am to the left side of my body. It seems like it might take some time for my two sides to get acquainted. . . ." There's a look on Fred's face that Pauline has never seen before. It's tender, almost shy. She flushes, sensing that Fred's internal shift is going to affect their friendship in an unexpected way. Confused, she seeks Margie's glance.

"There's all the time you need," Margie offers.

"Right," he says. "There's plenty of time. And I have a hunch there aren't just two homes either. There are probably lots of homes in between the old and new. Well, there's more work to do, but I feel freer already."

"You look freer too," Bill comments. "Good demonstration, Pauline."

"Thanks," Pauline replies, smiling and scooting over so Fred can join her on the couch. "That blending exploration certainly is powerful. You know, when I went through that process exploring my sitting position, I had a very scary feeling at one point. My pelvis felt too wide open. It was odd, because I was just sitting there on the piano bench. I felt like I was about eight years old."

Bill has been following the discussion with interest until now. He recognizes the feeling Pauline is describing, but it makes him feel uncomfortable to hear her talking about it so openly. He glances at his watch. Maybe he ought to go into the kitchen and warm up his coffee.

Margie and Fred are listening intently as Pauline continues her story. "Then Margie asked me, 'What did little Pauline need to know that you know now?' It was the perfect question, Margie. I went inside and explained to my little girl self about the birds and the bees, all the stuff that the boys at school were teasing the girls about, but that my mom thought I was too young to understand. She was never comfortable talking about sex. And I had an uncle who made inappropriate remarks. He was never physically abusive, but he used to tease me. It was all very confusing. As I reached puberty, I shut down the feelings in my body because I didn't understand them. And getting the explanations later on didn't make it safe to unlock those feelings. But when I talked with my younger self and explained things the way I wished they'd been explained back then, it made a huge difference in the way my body felt."

By this time Bill has retreated into the kitchen. Therapy has enabled him to talk more freely about himself with Kay, but such intimate sharing in a group, even though he is not doing the talking, is too much for him. The closeness and trust between the other three people is palpable. He can sense it, but he can't join in.

As Bill sits at the table stirring his coffee, he has a funny little daydream of Margie, Fred, Pauline, and him riding skateboards. They zip all around while he keeps falling off, still an awkward "stringbean." "Take a breath, old buddy," he counsels himself. "Feel the floor. . . ."

"Did you get what you need, Bill?" Margie sticks her head through the door.

"Sure did. These are great cookies. Did you make them?"

"Yes. There's lots more. Take some home to Kay if you'd like."

"Thanks."

"Listen. I noticed something about your structure when you walked out here. I'd like to share it with you."

"Okay, shoot."

"Well, to start with, you're a tall man."

"Now that's news!"

"What I mean is that doorways are too short for you. You had to duck your head to get in here. Did you know that?"

"I guess so. I'm used to it, though."

"Walk through the doorway again, Bill. Notice what you do."

Bill gets up and walks toward the living room. "I shrink my neck down into my chest, don't I?"

"Right. So what could you do instead?"

Bill walks back and forth a couple of times. He tries bending at the waist, tucking in his chin. In frustration, he pantomimes knocking a hole in the door frame.

Margie laughs. "Try bending your knees, silly."

He does. "Hey! They bend. They lower my height. What do you know!"

"Now you need to practice that a bit," says Margie. "You've been ducking your head for a long time, so every time you see a door, your nervous system tells you to duck. You've got to pattern a different response. You see a doorway, a little bell rings in your head, and your knees bend instead."

"Repetition is kind of like building a freeway, isn't it?"

"What do you mean?"

"Well, right now bending my knees when I see a door is just clearing a narrow trail. . . ."

"I get it." Margie smiles. "Yes, you have to turn it into an eight-lane highway."

When Margie and Bill rejoin the others, they find Fred standing in front of the fireplace with his eyes closed. "What's he doing?" Bill whispers to Pauline.

"You don't have to be quiet," Fred says. "I'm just getting a handle on these sensations so I can find them again."

"Try taking the feeling with you as you walk," Pauline suggests.

The others watch Fred as he paces around the room. "What just happened?" Margie asks at one point. "Whatever you were thinking or feeling just then sure made a difference in your walk."

"I was pretending that the floor was soft, like I was walking on thick, expensive carpet."

"Well, that made your feet articulate better, and your whole body suddenly looked more fluid. Any other impressions as you walk that way?"

"Yes. . . . It seems gentler, like it doesn't take so much will. Yes— less will." Fred looks slightly disconcerted.

"Great," Margie says. "Now go back to walking your old way and try blending. Walk with full-out will, then with no will, and then try some variations in between so you begin to find more choices."

"I want to try this too," Pauline says, kicking off her shoes.

Soon they're all marching and ambling around the apartment, bumping into each other, and finally laughing so hard they collapse on the floor.

"Would you be willing to try one more thing, Fred?" Margie asks, after the giggles have died down.

"Sure."

"Okay. Feel that relaxed, unforced state in your body. And now picture yourself at work. Weave just the right amount of that state into your work scene. Too much gentleness wouldn't get the job done. But a little bit could make it easier."

Fred nods.

"Now picture yourself working with the kids. How much of your new state of being is appropriate in that situation?"

Fred nods again.

"And picture something you want to be doing in the future. Imagine yourself doing it with just the right balance of force and gentleness."

After several minutes, Fred looks around. "I was thinking about my dream," he said. "You know, I'd like to start my own fitness center some day. A Gravity Game fitness center, where the instructors are trained in the principles we've been learning."

"Great idea," the others exclaim, almost in unison.

"I think so. But what I saw just now during that exercise was that I have to let my project develop from a balanced place in myself. If I force it, if I make it happen with my strong right arm, so to speak, then I'll be sabotaging the very thing I'm trying to accomplish."

"There's that path of simplicity again," Pauline says. "Seems like there's no end to gravity's common sense."

"Margie," Fred says, turning toward her and reaching out his hand to touch her shoulder. "You should be a therapist. You're really good at this, do you know that?"

"Oh," Margie sighs. Her face flushing, she starts to turn away. Then suddenly she's collapsed against Fred's chest, his arm around her as she lets the sobs come. Bill feels a weight on his shoulders and tension in his legs as if they'd like to be elsewhere. But this time he takes a deep breath, closes his eyes, and lets himself feel. Margie, much as she annoys him sometimes, is a good friend. He stays put.

"It's such a balancing act," Margie says when she can talk. "You know those acrobats in the circus, the ones who stand on each others' shoulders?"

The others nod.

"Well, the only way they stay balanced is by letting themselves be in motion. The guy on the bottom is riding a bicycle. If anybody tries to hold still, that's the end of it. And that's what I keep forgetting—that it's all a process. It's dynamic. But I keep trying to control it."

BALANCING YOUR
BODY

Her friends wait for Margie to complete her thoughts, sensing that she's struggling to free a part of herself that's been restrained for a long time.

"You see, I think I should be a therapist too. But when I think about all the training I'll need, then it seems like another mountain I have to climb. And I'm tired."

"What are you tired of, Marge?" asks Bill.

"For a long time now I've been helping everyone close to me keep it together. And people at work too. I'm tired of helping people! So what kind of a therapist would I be in that case?"

"Where do you feel that in your body?" Bill asks.

"Feel what?"

"The tension of helping and being tired from helping."

"Good question," Margie says. "Let's see, it's in my head. It's like a cap I'm wearing, tension all around my skull. And somewhere else . . . in my elbows. Yes. It's like always being ready to do something."

"Always being 'at arms'?"

"Yes. Ever ready."

"Well, let's deal with the cap first, okay?" Bill asks.

"Okay."

"What happens if you take off the cap?"

The group is quiet as they wait for Margie's answer. Fred and Pauline exchange glances, amazed at Bill's uncharacteristic audacity.

Margie is smiling now, crying and smiling at the same time. "If I stopped holding on to my head I could listen to my heart," she says. "It's that simple. And my heart would be irresponsible."

"How irresponsible could it be?"

"*Very* irresponsible!" Margie stands up and stretches. "And it would tell my head to turn around and take a look at the world." She rocks her body to and fro, arms swinging like branches in a strong wind. "Be a gypsy!" Margie is laughing now, her whole body loose. "This is crazy. I feel drunk!"

"And why not be a gypsy?"

"Because. . . ." She starts to straighten up.

"Because why?"

Margie frowns now and crosses her arms. "Because I'm too old to be tramping around the world like a hippie!"

"Now there's a stuck belief if I ever heard one," says Pauline.

"As if thirty-seven were a death sentence. And you! You're the one telling *me* to follow my dream."

"And me too," says Fred.

Margie considers it a while. "I guess I speak what I need to hear, don't I?"

"Want to try something, Marge?" Bill asks.

"Sure."

"Imagine yourself with 'round-the-world airfare and a passport in your pocket. Feel that possibility in every cell. Throw caution to the winds. You can help all those people when you get back. Go walk around a bit with *that* feeling in your body."

Margie disappears down the hall and returns wearing a jacket. "I'm sure you guys can do without me for a while. I'm taking my piece of the planet out for a stroll."

"We'll muddle along," Bill says, waving her out the door.

Half an hour later, Fred and Bill are playing Scrabble while Pauline amuses herself playing some old standards on the piano. Margie is still out, and the others are grateful for a break from the intense sharing. Once again, gravity has given them more than they bargained for.

"Oh! You startled me. How was your walk?" Margie has come in silently and stands listening to the music.

"I hiked up the hill. It's so crisp and clear—you can see all the stars. I feel lucky to live where it's still safe to take walks late at night."

Margie has an expression on her face that Pauline has never seen before. She looks a lot younger. "I think I'm going to do it, Paulie."

"What is it exactly that you want to do? I still don't really understand."

"I want to see the world, Paulie." She slides onto the bench beside her friend. "Travel. Just that. I've never talked about it because I never let myself really believe I could just take off. I have the money I've saved to buy a house. But what do I need with a house compared with the feeling of coming home to myself? You know, tonight I realized that I've been trying to be perfect at the Gravity Game. My head has been getting in the way again. But the minute I hold forth in my head, I destroy the freedom of my heart. And Fred's right, you know."

"About what?"

"About will. When I was walking up the hill, letting my heart guide my steps instead of my head, it was effortless. It's amazing how much excess will we use without even being aware of it. And it isn't just the physical ease, although my body does feel quite light. It's like a psychic weight has been lifted too. In this state I don't have to be ready for whatever might happen, because I'm present in the moment. Each moment."

"That sounds like freedom."

"The freedom of trusting the body."

The two women sit together at the piano for a while. It's been a full evening.

"Maybe we should call it a night," Margie says at last. "My eyelids are beginning to feel like lead."

"Time to cash in your chips, gentlemen," Pauline calls to the Scrabble players. "The womenfolk have had enough awareness for one evening."

"But what about the song you promised us? Hi, Marge. How was the walk?"

"Bill, that was incredible," Margie says, hugging him. "I can never thank you enough. And talk about being a therapist. Maybe you should give that some thought yourself."

"Well, I think I'm going to be too busy," Bill says, "being a dad."

"Bill!" they exclaim in unison, scrambling to embrace him.

"Talk about changes! This calls for a toast," Fred says, raising his coffee mug in the air. "To Dad!"

Bill's face is unusually ruddy as Pauline serenades him with a jazzy rendition of "My Heart Belongs to Daddy." Bill basks in the attention, letting a layer of his privacy fall away.

"This has been great, you guys," says Margie. "I wonder what our next reunion will bring?"

"How about a toast to the gypsy life!" says Bill.

"And a toast to gravity!" says Pauline.

"To *gravity!*" they echo.

Dancing with Gravity

And so the Gravity Gang lived more happily ever after than they might have otherwise, learning, as they did, that gravity is your partner, not your adversary. Certain prerequisite conditions helped the four friends make their discoveries. They were open-minded, courageous, and honest with themselves, and willing for their lives to change in response to changes in their bodies. And they had each other, a network of supportive and interested friends. I hope their stories have helped you develop a curiosity about how gravity might impact *your* life.

Remember the Christmas star, the symbol that unites gravity and love? Suppose you could stand on that star, a few light years down the road, and look back at the movements of your life right now. You'd be too far away to hear the music, but you could watch the dance—the moving shapes and rhythms of your body. What feelings would the choreography of your life convey?

I hope this book has given you some tools for enhancing your choreography and has drawn your attention to your power and responsibility as choreographer. Ultimately, your relationship to gravity is not a game. It's a dance; and a metaphor for love.

INSTITUTES FOR STRUCTURAL BODYWORK AND BODY/MIND THERAPY

Listed below are addresses and information on goals and approaches of various institutes for structural bodywork and body/mind therapy. These institutes train practitioners to facilitate personal transformation through physically oriented exploration. Should you feel the need for trained support through your process, you can contact any of these organizations for information on practitioners in your area.

The Alexander Technique

The North American Society of Teachers of the Alexander
   Technique (NASTAT)
P.O. Box 3992
Champaign, IL 61826-3992
(217) 358-3529

Self-discovery and relief of physical tension through reeducation of the kinesthetic sense. Emphasis on conscious release of unnecessary muscle tension. Gentle touch and verbal suggestions guide the student in becoming aware of harmful postural patterns, inhibiting them and replacing them with beneficial habits.

Aston Patterning®

Aston Patterning®
P.O. Box 3568
Incline Village, NV 89450
(702) 831–8228

A process of unraveling the layers of tension stored in the body to allow the individual more freedom and comfort. Gentle bodywork, movement education, and environmental scrutiny are combined to help the client achieve alignment that best suits his or her own individual structure and needs.

Bodynamic Analysis

Bodynamic Institute/USA
P.O. Box 6008
Albany, CA 94706-6008
(510) 524-8090

A somatic developmental psychotherapy based on the correlation each muscle has with its corresponding psychological function. The work includes building ego structure by working with undeveloped skills and impulses. This empowers adults in their daily lives and builds the resources necessary for resolving childhood trauma.

Body-Mind Centering™

The School for Body-Mind Centering™
189 Pondview Drive
Amherst, MA 01002
(413) 256-8615

An experiential study based on anatomical, physiological, psychological, and developmental movement principles, leading to an understanding of how the mind expresses itself through movement. Internal focus and gentle hands-on work help students to explore the physical and emotional expression inherent in different body systems and to repattern movements and mind.

Continuum

Continuum Studio
c/o Emilie Conrad-Da'oud
1629 18th Street, Studio #7
Santa Monica, CA 90404
(310) 453-4402

Experiencing the essential, intrinsic movements of the body to facilitate healing and creativity. Private and group sessions provide a context in which students develop sensitivity to the subtle movements of life, from breath and the fluid movement of tissue to patterns of interactions with others.

The Feldenkrais Method

The Feldenkrais Guild
524 Ellsworth Street
P.O. Box 489
Albany, OR 97321-0143
(503) 926-0981

Subconscious holding patterns are brought to awareness and released, in an effort to reclaim our natural body-brain integration. Education is based on the student's sense of rightness rather than working toward a specific structural ideal. Gentle manipulation, inward-focused attention, and nonstrenuous movements retrain the mind and body to more efficient patterns of expression.

Hakomi Therapy

Hakomi Institute
1800 30th Street, Suite 201
Boulder, CO 80301
(303) 443-6209

Transformational work grounded in gentleness, mindful awareness, and respect for the mind-body continuum. Behavior, body structure, and physiology are influenced by the exploration of deeply held beliefs, guiding images, and early memories. Communication at the interface of mind and body assists the client to access his/her own self-healing capacity and inner wisdom.

Hellerwork

Hellerwork
406 Berry Street
Mt. Shasta, CA 96067
(800) 392-3900, (916) 926-2500

Enhanced body consciousness through balancing the body in gravity. Deep-tissue massage combined with movement reeducation and dialogue on emotional themes assists the client in achieving harmony between body and self.

Neuro Linguistic Programming (NLP)

Dynamic Learning Center
P.O. Box 1112
Ben Lomond, CA 95005
(408) 336-3457

Individual counseling and problem solving based on increasing the flexibility of the way experience is coded in the mind. Personal change is checked for physical ecology and integration. Group seminars and trainings facilitate personal transformation.

Process Work

Process Work Center of Portland
733 N.W. Everett
Box 11/Suite 3C
Portland, OR 97209
(503) 223-8188

Individual counseling emphasizes the interrelationship of physical, psychological, and transpersonal experiences. The signals found within individual suffering are explored for solutions to problems and strategies for healing and personal growth. Group seminars and trainings foster individual growth.

Rolfing® and Rolfing Movement

The Rolf Institute
302 Pearl Street, P.O. Box 1868
Boulder, CO 80306-1868
(800) 530-8875, (303) 449-5903

In Rolfing, deep tissue massage and movement education release the body's structure from lifelong patterns of tension, permitting gravity to realign it. The experience of physical balance leads to enhanced self-image and personal evolution. Rolfing Movement employs gentle touch, guided awareness, and verbal dialogue to assist the student in replacing physical tensions and their concurrent emotions with free and well-integrated movement.

Structural Awareness

Nolte System of Movement Education
Dorothy Nolte, Ph.D.
24651 Via Raza
Lake Forest, CA 92630
(714) 380-9467

Movement education to improve physical alignment and self-concept through awakening the body to patterns directed by gravity. Specific movement patterns, breathing, and imagery increase flexibility and free the body from old habits.

Structural Integration

Guild for Structural Integration, Inc.
P. O. Box 1559
Boulder, CO 80306
(800) 447-0150, (303) 447-0122

Deep tissue massage and movement education release the body's structure from lifelong patterns of tension, permitting gravity to realign it. The experience of physical balance leads to enhanced self-image and personal evolution.

The Trager Approach

Trager Institute
33 Millwood
Mill Valley, CA 94941
(415) 388-2688

Facilitates release of psycho-physiological patterns that block freedom of movement. Client's body is rhythmically moved by the practioner producing deep relaxation and release of a mental and physical stresses. A dancelike sequence of movements can be practiced to enhance and continue the process. Structural and functional improvements occur spontaneously as a result of this sensory repatterning.

BIBLIOGRAPHY

Andreas, Connirae, and Steve Andreas. *Heart of the Mind: Engaging Your Inner Power to Change with Neuro Linguistic Programming.* Moab, Utah: Real People Press, 1989.

Bandler, Richard, and John Grinder. *Frogs Into Princes: Neuro Linguistic Programming.* Moab, Utah: Real People Press, 1979.

Barlow, Wilfred. *The Alexander Technique: How to Use Your Body Without Stress.* Rochester, Vt.: Healing Arts Press, 1991.

Bertherat, Therese, and Carol Bernstein. *The Body Has Its Reasons.* Rochester, Vt.: Healing Arts Press, 1989.

Dychtwald, Ken. *Bodymind.* Los Angeles: J. P. Tarcher, 1986.

Fahey, Brian W. *The Power of Balance: A Rolfing View of Health.* Portland, Oreg.: Metamorphous Press, 1989.

Feldenkrais, Moshe. *Awareness Through Movement: Health Exercises for Personal Growth.* San Francisco: Harper San Francisco, 1972.

Gendlin, Eugene T. *Focusing.* Third Edition. New York: Bantam Books, 1982.

Houston, Jean. *The Possible Human: A Course in Extending Your Physical, Mental, and Creative Abilities.* Los Angeles, J. P. Tarcher, 1982.

Hunt, Valerie, W. Massey, R. Weinberg, R. Bruyere, and P. Hahn. *A Study of Structural Integration from Neuromuscular, Energy, Field, and Emotional Approaches.* Unpublished Report (UCLA), 1977.

Keleman, Stanley. *Emotional Anatomy*. Berkeley, Calif.: Center Press, 1985.

Kurtz, Ron. *Body-Centered Psychotherapy: The Hakomi Method*. Mendocino, Calif.: LifeRhythm, 1980.

———, and Hector Prestera. *The Body Reveals: An Illustrated Guide to the Psychology of the Body*. New York: Harper & Row, 1976.

Lee, Jennette. *This Magic Body*. New York: Viking, 1946.

Masters, Robert, and Jean Houston. *Listening to the Body*. New York: Dell, 1989.

Mindell, Arnold. *Coma: Key to Awakening*. Boston: Shambhala, 1989.

———. *Working with the Dreaming Body*. London: Routledge & Kegan, Paul, 1985.

Pierce, Alexandra, and Roger Pierce. *Expressive Movement: Posture and Action in Daily Life, Sports, and the Performing Arts*. New York: Plenum Press, 1989.

———. *Generous Movement: A Practical Guide to Balance in Action*. Redlands, Calif.: The Center of Balance Press, 1991.

Rolf, Ida P. *Gravity, An Unexplored Factor In a More Human Use of Human Beings*. Pamphlet. Boulder, Co.: Rolf Institute, 1979.

———. *Rolfing and Physical Reality*. Rochester, Vt.: Healing Arts Press, 1990.

———. *Rolfing: Reestablishing the Natural Alignment and Structural Integration of the Human Body for Vitality and Well-Being*. Rochester, Vt.: Healing Arts Press. 1989.

Todd, Mable E. *The Thinking Body: A Study of the Balancing Forces of Dynamic Man*. New York: Dance Horizons, 1968.

INDEX

BOOKS OF RELATED INTEREST